THE POLITICAL LIFE OF SENSATION

DUKE UNIVERSITY PRESS

DURHAM AND LONDON

2009

The Political Life of Sensation

DAVIDE PANAGIA

DUKE UNIVERSITY PRESS

Printed in the United States

of America on acid-free paper ∞

Designed by C. H. Westmoreland

Typeset in Dante by Keystone Typesetting, Inc.

Library of Congress Cataloging-in-Publication

Data appear on the last printed

page of this book.

PER LISANNA

The number of the senses is not fewer than six.

JEAN ANTHELME BRILLAT-SAVARIN,
The Physiology of Taste

CONTENTS

ILLUSTRATIONS

GRAZIE

I owe much of what is included in these pages to the encounters and conversations with scholars and artists operating at the intersections of theory, culture, politics, and aesthetics.

In this regard I extend my first note of gratitude to Marco Orlandi, whose restoration of the Liberty Edicola (newsstand) in Casalmaggiore, Italy, as well as his reflections on the ethical, political, and aesthetic dimensions of cultural preservation proved invaluable to my own considerations. Not to be overlooked are the people of Casalmaggiore themselves and, most notably, mayor Luciano Toscani, Carlo Gardani, and the gracious staff of the Biblioteca Civica A. E. Mortara—especially Sandra Furini and Vittorio Rizzi—for their research expertise and their permission to reproduce some of the archival material in these pages. I would also like to thank Luigi Briselli for his technical know-how in providing reproductions of archival photographs. Last but not least, I thank the friends at the Fuori Porta (Cappella, CR) who cultivate a unique space of *convivium* and restoration.

As always, my writing and ideas are indebted to the critical interventions of friends who share my passion regarding the relationship between aesthetics and politics. First among these is Bill Connolly, whose generosity and intellectual creativity are a persistent source of challenge, learning, and encouragement. I learn more than I can process from the writings of Jacques Rancière, and to him I am grateful for the time he regularly takes out of his busy schedule to discuss my work and ideas. Mort Schoolman's enthusiasm about the aesthetic dimensions of democratic life is contagious. I thank him for sharing with me the originality of his work and insights, and for his support.

I consider myself fortunate to have intellectual camaraderies throughout the world. For their hospitality and attention to my work, I thank the research consortium of Vincenzo Cesareo, Mauro Magatti, Arpad Szakolczai, and Italo Vaccarini of the Sociology department at the Università Cattolica del Sacro Cuore di Milano. I also extend much gratitude to Arash Abizadeh, Amanda Anderson, Mary Bellhouse, Cristina Beltrán, Jane Bennett, Roger Berkowitz, Mark Canuel, Bill Chaloupka, Drucilla Cornell, Jodi Dean, Michael Dillon, Lisa Disch, Thomas Dumm, Konrad Eisenbichler, Frances Ferguson, Kennan Ferguson, Michaele Ferguson, Joshua Foa Dienstag, Jason Frank, Nancy Fraser, Robert Hariman, Bonnie Honig, Steve Johnston, Jennet Kirkpatrick, Nikolas Kompridis, Sharon Krause, Arthur Kroker, John Louis Lucaites, Erin Manning, Robyn Marasco, Patchen Markell, Lori Marso, Brian Massumi, Dean Mathiowetz, Kirstie McClure, John McCormick, Laurie Naranch, Anne Norton, Peter Nyers, Paul Patton, Riccardo Pelizzo, Elisabetta Povoledo, Guido Pugliese, Olga Zorzi Pugliese, John D. Rockefeller V, Kam Shapiro, Michael Shapiro, Steven Shaviro, Jon Howard Simons, Verity Smith, Gabrielle Spiegel, Dan Stone, Tracy Strong, Lucas Swaine, Christina Tarnopolsky, Ananya Vajpeyi, Paul Vogt, Stephen White, Elizabeth Wingrove, Linda Zerilli, and Karen Zivi. I thank you all for your friendship and critical engagement.

The Cultural Studies Department and the Centre for the Study of Theory, Culture, and Politics at Trent University are exciting places for interdisciplinary research, and much of my work was facilitated by the collaborative research clusters that gather around the Canada Research Chair in Cultural Studies Media Research Lab at the Principal's Lodge of Traill College. Here I have had the good fortune to find colleagues who encourage me to explore forms of inquiry that I had previously not considered. In this regard, I am particularly grateful to Emilia Angelova, Zsuzsa Baross, Costas Boundas, Richard Dellamora, Victoria de Zwaan, Charmaine Eddy, Betsy Ermarth, John

Fekete, Bernie Hodgson, David Holdsworth, Veronica Hollinger, Ihor Junyk, Ian McLachlan, David Morris, James Penney, Elaine Stavro, Doug Torgerson, and Andrew Wernick. Another good fortune about being at Trent is having great students. Specifically, I would like to thank two graduate students—Jo Anne Colson and Katharine Wolfe—for teaching me a great deal about politics and aesthetics. I am also grateful to my research assistant, Tim Hanafin, who helped with the technical production of this manuscript in numerous ways. Last but not least, I would like to acknowledge the exceptional administrative assistance of Jeannine Crowe and Nancy Legate.

Courtney Berger of Duke University Press demonstrated, once again, her intelligence, skill, and talent at every level of the editorial process. In this regard, I am also indebted to the excellent critical comments provided by two blind reviewers of Duke University Press.

Dulcis in fundo I thank my family and, especially, my wife Lisanna. To her strength, courage, and love I dedicate this book. To my mother Marisa, my brother Marcello, and to Cesare, Carla, Silvia, Fabio, Birgit, Edoardo, Ludovica, Vittoria, and Giulia I am grateful for the unconditional joy, care, and support they give me.

Previous versions of the prologue were presented at the "Democratic Aesthetics" research seminar organized by Jon Howard Simons at the 2007 meeting of the National Communication Association (Chicago, Ill.) as well as at the Università Cattolica del Sacro Cuore (Milano). Versions of chapter 1 were presented at the "Gilles Deleuze: Image and Text" conference (Columbia, S.C., 2007), at the 2007 meeting of the American Political Science Association (Chicago, Ill.), and at the New School for Social Research Political Theory Colloquium. Various incarnations of chapter 2 were presented at the "City Limits?" conference (Winnipeg, MB, 2004), the Western Political Science Association (Oakland, Calif., 2005), the Toronto Renaissance and Reformation Colloquium (2005), and the Montreal Political Theory Workshop (2005). A version of chapter 3 was presented at the 2005 Renaissance Society of America conference (Cambridge, UK). A previous iteration of chapter 4 was presented at the 2006 meeting of the

Western Political Science Association (Albuquerque, N. Mex.) and originally appeared as "The Effects of Viewing: Caravaggio, Bacon, and *The Ring*" in *Theory and Event* 10:4. Used by permission of the publisher. Chapter 5 was presented at the Trent University Philosophy Society (Peterborough, Canada), the 2007 Canadian Society for Italian Studies International Conference (Trieste, Italy), and "The Politics of Food, Taste, and Time" panel of the 2006 meeting of the American Political Science Association (Philadelphia, Pa.). A special note of gratitude goes to Werlen Hansjakob, the Philadelphia Slow Food Convivium leader, for providing victuals for that event. Chapter 5 also appeared as "You're Eating Too Fast! On Disequality and an Ethos of Convivium" in the *Journal for Cultural Research* 11:3, reprinted here by permission of the publisher. I thank all the members of these audiences for their attention and active participation.

The research presented in this book could not have been possible without the generous institutional and financial support of the Canada Research Chairs Program and a Social Sciences and Humanities Research Council of Canada Standard Research Grant.

PROLOGUE

Narratocracy and the Contours of Political Life

> The distinction between touch and sight are unknown in primordial perception. It is only as a result of the science of the body that we learn to distinguish between our senses. MAURICE MERLEAU-PONTY

There is nothing quite like the sensation that accompanies an idea. The idea doesn't have to be particularly sophisticated, or even elaborate. It can be as simple as figuring out exactly the right gift to give someone for his or her birthday, or how to respond to a challenging essay question. But when it strikes you, it invades your life. All of a sudden, something that didn't have either shape or texture begins to take form. You read a phrase and think "*les mots justes!*" Or you come across an image in a recipe book, a movie, or a YouTube video and exclaim "it's perfect!" The idea affects you at diverse registers of experience: It has a sound, you can see it, touch it, taste it, and sometimes even smell it. Connections are drawn that hadn't occurred to you, and you become convinced of the concreteness of your thought formation. Something as vaporous and ethereal as a rumination is transformed into a palpable representation, and you allow yourself to experience, not only the material impact of that representation, but also the intensity that accompanies the transformation itself. In short, you are captured by an appearance and the indeterminable conviction that accompanies the moment of capture that transects you. *The Political Life of Sensation* explores these dimensions of aesthetic experience and their political potential.

Such experiences, though frequent, are short lived because the intensity of the moment passes rather quickly. We are also suspicious of them: these are experiences about particular things that often don't make sense to us, or at the very least if the sensation persists, we try to make sense of it by fitting it into some kind of context or overarching life-schema. Speaking nonsense, for instance, is perceived as an unwelcome failure that needs to be overcome with better thinking, more deliberation, and the kind of storytelling that will help make sense of the world and justify our place in it. But the thing about the activity of sense making is that it always takes sense itself for granted; we always already know the shape and sound an utterance must have in order for it to have meaning or to count as political speech; we are never really content in addressing nonsense as we rarely feel comfortable with its disruptions. And yet, moments of sensation punctuate our everyday existence, and in doing so, they puncture our received wisdoms and common modes of sensing.

In this book I examine ways in which sensation interrupts common sense. By sensation I mean neither sense nor perception (though both are crucially involved), but rather the heterology of impulses that register on our bodies without determining a body's nature or residing in any one organ of perception. In this respect, I consider sensation to be an experience of unrepresentability in that a sensation occurs without having to rely on a recognizable shape, outline, or identity to determine its value. Though we may not have fixed strategies for representing a sensation, we can invent or configure ways of relating the experience it affords (assuming we decide it's an experience worth relating). The limits posed by sensation's unrepresentability thus interrupt our conventional ways of perceiving the world and giving it value. I argue that such moments of interruption (or what I will variously call disarticulation or disfiguration) are political moments because they invite occasions and actions for reconfiguring our associational lives. My ambition in these pages is to examine the forces of interruption and reconfiguration that, I argue, comprise the aesthetico-political dimensions of democratic life.

Politics happens when a relation of attachment or detachment is formed between heterological elements: it is a part-taking in the activities of representation that renders perceptible what had previously been insensible.[1] When chocolate bakers leave their shops to enact public displays of chocolate preparation in the piazzas of Italy in order to protest the standardization of taste by the European community (see chapter 2), a convergence of heterological elements ensues (i.e., the bakers, the chocolate, the piazzas, the passersby, the mouth) that renders perceptible a new political subjectivity: the tasting subject.[2] Flavor—not speech—turns the mouth into an organ of political action, and the piazza is transformed into a space for taste. This potential simultaneity of dissimilars is the irrational truth of democratic life. We think that contrarieties cannot coexist unless they are made compatible; yet democratic politics perseveres in its insistence that any two or more people, groups, images, identities, subjectivities, and so forth, can persist simultaneously. One could go so far as to suggest that heterology is the ontological condition of democratic politics.

But before such political relations may be forged, before things are rendered perceptible, an interruption of previous forms of relating occurs. This book examines the dynamics of such interruptions when there is a disarticulation of our organoleptic correspondences.[3] With this in mind, *The Political Life of Sensation* is also about the activities of disfiguration and reconfiguration of the sensible. By "sensible" I mean both "what makes sense" and "what can be sensed." Though most of us live our lives with the confidence that things, values, and other lives circulate around us with some continuity, we nonetheless also experience moments of breakdown, when the certitudes of circulation collapse. These moments can be at once tragic or comic, fill us with despair or pleasure, give us insight or distract our trains of thought. Whatever the case may be, they are moments that exceed the limits that structure our daily living, and they interrupt the assurances that guarantee the slumber of subjectivity. They are for these reasons ethical moments, not because they are rule bound or normative, but because they compel us to relinquish our attachments and acknowledge that our subjectivities are inconsistent and open to repetitions of articulation. They are instances of what Michel Foucault refers to as *ethopoetic* forms of knowledge "concerning things, the world, the gods and men, but whose effect and function are to change the subject's being."[4]

Aesthetic theory and criticism are central to our appreciation of such ethopoetic moments, especially as they relate to questions of judgment: how can we give value to an object when we lack confidence in our bannisters of judgment?[5] What, in other words, accounts for our convictions if the disjunctive work of sensation denies us recourse to a belief, motivation, or norm that might justify our appraisals? These are central questions of modern aesthetics since the appearance of Kant's third critique, and I also consider them as central to contemporary democratic theory: that is, a principal dilemma of any multicultural democratic society is to have to address how the pluralization of values within any one polity interrupts the ordered divisions that hold those polities together. Rather than developing normative arguments to resolve these questions, however, I turn to the writings on aesthetic reflection by a variety of contemporary and historical authors.

Many writers with diverse theoretical ambitions and orientations have struggled with some of the problems that I also grapple with in these pages. Given this, I should affirm at the outset that though I am indebted to, and have learned a great deal from, the work of psychoanalytic theorists who discuss the relationship between subjectivity, sensation, and appearances, I do not engage that tradition of critical thought in these pages.[6] Rather I move away from the ambition to interpret the meaning of objects and events and explore the developments of some recent scholarship in cultural theory that challenge the hermeneutic assumption that things must be meaningful in order to count as valuable (as if meaning were a property of the object described). Importantly, such hermeneutic efforts do provide us with strategies for signification, but, to echo Brian Massumi's critical interventions, "signifying gestures make sense,"[7] and it is not so much the making of sense as the interruption of sense that I explore in this book.

To be more precise, in the chapters that follow I engage potential sites of the dislocation of subjectivity in popular culture and the occasions of reconfiguration that such dislocations invite. I take this to be important political work done on a quotidian basis by groups and individuals, and it is work that takes place beneath and beyond the discursive register of communicative sense making. The disarticulation of the subject is a theory of action that looks to acts of disfiguration and reconfiguration as ways of—as Hannah Arendt says—"breaking fresh ground and acting without precedents."[8] But before the breaking of ground, before the imaginative acts of reconfiguration, there is the dissensus of sensation that disrupts our confidence in the correspondence between perception and signification.

The aesthetic and political concerns that motivate my inquiries stem from what I take to be a notable fact of pluralist democratic societies: namely, that individuals or groups in these societies attend to one another at the level of appearances. One of the important contributions that cultural theory has made to contemporary explorations in political thought is to highlight the extent to which political life is fundamentally a perceptual enterprise.[9] No less has this been the case with the critical insights of a variety of feminist theorists who examine the relationship between bodily experience, perception, and subjectivity.[10] In the following pages, I exploit these contributions that address the theory-culture-politics nexus by bringing to bear upon the dynamics of multicultural politics various accounts of perception, especially as regards the complexity of visuality in political life.[11]

If this might seem like an odd point of departure, consider how, at a crucial point in his study on the politics of recognition, Charles Taylor claims the following: "the demand for recognition [in political societies] is now explicit . . . [and] thanks to this idea, misrecognition has now graduated to the rank of a harm that can be hardheadedly enumerated."[12] Echoing Frantz Fanon, he concludes that one of the chief political tools employed by those in power is the deployment of images of peoples and cultures for the purpose of subjugation.[13] The fascinating thing about this claim is neither its accuracy nor its verifiability but, more importantly, its adoption of a theory of visual perception that remains dangling and unexplored. What Taylor and other admirers and critics of multiculturalism alike rely on is an account of how images work—how they circulate, how they transmit their appearances as multisensory phenomena, and how individuals acquire those sensations—without ever making that account explicit. In short, the "harm that can be hardheadedly enumerated" of multicultural politics assumes a regime of perception that informs public judgments of recognition and equality. Multicultural politics, we are left to conclude, is a politics of visuality.

This account of visual culture relies on a figurative conception of the image.[14] Taylor's concern in these passages (and in his work on multiculturalism more generally) isn't so much that individual or group images are valuable and ought to be respected; it is, rather, that their value is determined by their semantic content and that that meaning is available by pointing to a context.[15] However, in this story of the subjugating power of the image, very little attention, if any, is paid to the role of sensation and the forms of political reflection that make these appearances visible, that allow for us to turn our attentions to them, and in doing so enable us to be captured and convinced by them; that is, little attention is paid to the regimes of perception that ensure the political valence of an image.

Jacques Rancière calls such regimes of perception "partitions of the sensible."[16] By "partitions of the sensible" he does not simply mean that an aesthetic attunement to the world of politics shows us that there are different perspectives or points of view that must be recognized. On the contrary, Rancière's phrase suggests that our modes of perceiving the world, of sensing the presence of others, are parsed; that as subjects of perception, human beings are partial creatures variously divided. A partition of the sensible thus refers to perceptual forms of knowledge that parse what is and is not sensible, what counts as making (i.e., fabricating) sense and what is available to be sensed.[17] "Politics," Rancière thus concludes, "is an activity of reconfiguration of that which is given to the sensible."[18]

These dynamics of the sensible suggest that our capacity to comprehend things is grounded in a particular organoleptic configuration that constitutes the self-evident dispositions of a sensing body: we always already know what it means to sense, what seeing, touching, and hearing are. Such assurances and the practices of sense making that enable them are, by definition, political. They relate our bodies to the world, but also determine the conditions through and by which we might sense the world and those who occupy it; in short, such regimes of perception confer what counts as common sense. But, we might ask, what if the relationship between our sensory organs and acts of perception is not as certain as we presume?

Consider the case of skin, the first threshold of touch. To touch, as Erin Manning has recently suggested, "is to conceive of a simultaneity that requires the courage to face the in-between."[19] There is no impermeable boundary that our skin might guarantee, and yet we insist on perceiving skin as a containment vessel. Gender, race, sex, desire, beauty, weight, and height are signifiers that correspond to the experience of skin as a determinate organ of perception. So it is that with skin we have a partition of the sensible that guarantees a series of other equivalences like recognition, impermeability, unity, and cohesiveness that are transcribed onto our political conceptions of individuality, identity, and subjectivity and work to overcome skin's fluidity and porosity.

What would happen if our senses of skin were interrupted and we experienced skin as an organ of disfiguration? What if we went even further and stopped thinking organically so that the shape of our bodies was no longer determined by the disposition of our organs? Skin might stop being a determinate organ of perception and could become a nodule of sensation: my finger touches your arm and you can at once see, hear, and smell my touch. Therein lies sensation. For a brief moment, I alter my disposition toward you, and yours toward me. Now we have a new and temporary partition of the sensible whose durational intensity reconfigures our postures of perceptual attention without requiring that such a new configuration become either a precedent, rule, or expectation.[20]

Some current research in the field of neuroaesthetics (a branch of neuroscience) also examines such assumptions about judgment, perception, and the forms of attention we give the world of appearances. A recent study in *Nature Neuroscience*, for instance, shows that our eyes are in constant motion, even when focusing on a single object. Every three seconds, our visual field shifts without our being aware of it: we have the impression of fixed perception but that sense of stability is in tension with our physical eye movements, or saccades. Thus we lose up to fifteen percent of perceived temporal experience because we cannot process the rapidity with which our eye movement registers the external world. In short, we all seem to suffer from a version of attention deficit as there exists a three-second interval between eye movement and the attention we give to objects in our field of vision. "As eye movement and attention are known to be tightly related," these researchers explain, "it is worthwhile to consider the possible role of attention in temporal compression. Attention is known to influence perceived duration and also temporal order."[21] But this kind of eye movement also suggests an opposite effect, "a general dampening of attention at the time of saccades, a time when information is least reliable."[22]

The dampening of attention and the subsequent unreliability of information that results from the relationship between eye movement, visuality, and registered perception does not describe a cognitive failure. It is, rather, an account of two distinct sequences of perceptual focus—the outline and the contour—that, as Maurice Merleau-Ponty explained some years ago, were also crucial to Paul Cézanne's explorations in painting.[23] The uniqueness of Cézanne's work for Merleau-Ponty is its ability to move beyond impressionism and depict objects "as they appear to instantaneous perception, without fixed contours bound together by light and air."[24] By developing a color technique that uses warm colors and blacks to depict the gradual formation of objects on a canvas, Cézanne breaks with impressionism and also breaks with the necessity of using outlines to draw shapes. "In giving up the outline," Merleau-Ponty explains, "Cézanne was abandoning himself to the chaos of sensations, which would upset the objects and constantly suggest illusions, as, for example the illusion we have when we move our head that the objects themselves are moving—if our judgment did not constantly set the appearances straight."[25]

Merleau-Ponty's distinction between judgment (straight appearances) and sensation (illusion and chaos) invoked to describe Cézanne's works relies on the distinction between an outline and a contour which rests on the even more basic distinction between a "primordial," or lived, perception and geometry.[26] Rather than painting a pure impression, Cézanne painted the experience of sensation, and the difference between the two efforts rests on the difference between painting objects by outlining shapes and using overlapping tones to create contours. "If one outlines the shape of an apple," Merleau-Ponty clarifies, "one makes an object of the shape, whereas the contour is rather the ideal limit towards which the sides of the apple recede in depth."[27] The recognition of an apple, in other words, requires accepting the outline's capacity to give shape to objects. In contrast, a contour does not depict an apple but allows for the apple's appearance to emerge through the blurring of overlapping color tones. "That is why Cézanne follows the swelling of the object in modulated colors and indicates several outlines in blue. Rebounding among these, one's glance captures a shape that emerges from them all, just as it does in perception."[28]

To the extent that politics refers to the activity of rendering perceptible heterological elements, the insights that Merleau-Ponty offers regarding Cézanne's works help us appreciate how political life is comprised of the constant articulation and disarticulation of contours; and these kinds of activities are as informed by our aesthetic sensibilities as they are by our political ones. My inquiry into the political life of sensation thus stems from the following assumption: that the first political act is also an aesthetic one, a partitioning of sensation that divides the body and its organs of sense perception and assigns to them corresponding capacities for the making of sense. With sensation we enter a world of contours, resonances, vibrations, attunements, syntonizations, hapticities, and impulses, as Gilles Deleuze explains in his studies on painting.[29] Sensation is, as I suggested earlier, an interruption of sense; but it is important that we not reduce sensation to an objective achievement. An acknowledgment of sensation is, at best, a modest accomplishment because the moment of sensation is an unexpected moment of dampened attention, when one loses recourse to the networks, practices, and relays of attachment that sustain representation.

To address these concerns, I proceed by means of what I call a genealogy of political reflection. I use the term "political reflection" to describe the thought-activity that accompanies the ethopoetic dimensions of sensation. My use of this term is indebted to Merleau-Ponty's claim that "reflection obscures what we thought was clear. We believe we know what feeling, seeing, and hearing were, and now these words raise problems,"[30] and further, that reflection "knows itself as reflection-on-an-unreflective-experience, and consequently as a change in structure of our existence."[31] Reflection, as I understand it, is a modality of somacognition—of body thinking—that is oriented toward the indeterminacies that persist in political life. As the Italian architect Giovanni Garroni has recently written, "what is indeterminate in objects constitutes that ambiguous boundary that permits superimposition, allusion and even confusion. Instability is what subtracts objects from the solitude to which they would be condemned by a hypothetical absolute precision."[32]

A genealogy of political reflection is attentive to the ways in which individuals relate to indeterminacy and ambiguity and through that relation constitute themselves as subjects of perception. This, for instance, is what I find especially captivating about the attention to taste that the practitioners of Slow Food endorse. As I discuss in chapter 5, the eating of a Narragansett turkey becomes, for the journalist Michael Pollan, an experience of convivium that rearticulates his perceptions of gratitude. The ability to perceive something is not, in this formulation, an accomplishment that marks a kind of unveiling or illumination; it refers, rather, to the ways in which the postures of attention we occupy—the bendings of the frames of our bodies, the turnings of our heads, the raisings of our eyes, the pricking of our ears, and the opening of our mouths—are acts of ethical reconfiguration; they are part of the work we do on ourselves that allows us to live in, and endure, the impact of appearances. The turning of one's self is a relinquishing of our self that creates an ethical relationship with that from which we turn and with that toward which we turn; it is, in short, an ethical practice of *attending to* the world of appearances.

Thus, it is not at all obvious that at the moment of an appearance, of the emergence of a new political subjectivity, there will be conventions in place that will allow us to recognize the identity of the subject in question. Though we are affronted by a new appearance and face up to a political subjectivity's contour, at the moment of encounter recognition is an inadequate ethical response. The event of appearance is also an event of sensation and, as such, it is a disjunctive event that disarticulates the regimes of perception which allow us to establish the identity of an appearance. Rather than recognition, then, we have recourse to an act of admission: an appearance advenes upon us and we admit to it. But, as I explain in the epilogue to this book, such adveniences also invite reflection on an ethics of appearance, on those moments when we encounter and attend to an image but cannot fully account for it. Nor can we be sure that a discourse of accountability will help us in making sense of such an encounter because at the moment of impact, at the moment when an appearance advenes and we orient our postures of attention to it, we cannot confirm the outline or identity of the composition in question. The appearance of a new political subjectivity, like the appearance of an image, invites a relinquishing and a reconfiguring of our selves. Such reconfigurations, I submit, are ethical acts of part-taking in the political life of sensation.

On Narratocracy

In the following pages I bring to bear some recent reflections in aesthetics and cultural theory on the writings of selected historical and contemporary political thinkers. What I offer are not complete or comprehensive readings of any one thinker, theme, artifact, or event. Rather, I portray partial moments of engagement that help pose questions regarding the dynamics of aesthetics and politics. In this regard, a principal site of concern in the following pages is the privileging of narrative as a genre for the exposition of claims and ideas in contemporary political thought, or what I call *narratocracy*.

Narratocracy is a prevailing regime of perception in the theoretical analysis of political phenomena. It offers the narrative line which is the story line that determines the trajectory of an action, but it is also the stenographic mark that traces a figure (of speech, of thought, of script, etc.) across a blank page; it is an outline that renders an object, event, practice, or person at once visible and available for accountability. This is what it means to delineate or give an account of something, and this "giving an account" orients the perceptibility of an appearance and our postures of attention to it. The story line thus incises itself onto a field of vision and begins the work of conviction. Narratocracy, or the rule of narrative, is the organization of a perceptual field according to the imperative of rendering things readable.

Narratocracy refers both to the governance of narrative as a standard for the expression of ideas and to the rules that parse the perceptual field according to what is and is not valuable action, speech, or thought. That an event may be rendered readable thus gives it a value and enables its mediatic circulation and access to the conditions that constitute its political legitimacy. Much can be said about this readerly repose of political thought, as Hannah Arendt does by first defining politics as a space of appearance and then committing those appearances to an Aristotelian *poiesis* of *muthos* (emplotment).[33] But by insisting on their narrative qualities, we condition appearances to the perceptual expectations of readability, situating them within a system of visibility and sayability that insists on their capacity to make sense. "Contraries," Michel de Certeau explains, "are therefore compatible within the same text under the condition that it is narrative. Temporalization creates the possibility of making coherent an order and its 'heteroclite', its irregularity."[34] In short, our ability to generate story lines determines our representational skills as well as our specific capacities for making sense of the heterology of political life.

Narratocracy commits vision to readerly sight while partitioning the body into specific areas of sensory competency. That is, our relation to "account giving" qua storytelling, and the narratocratic postures of visual attention that accompany this, are enabled by "an organization of the visible"[35] that directs an individual's turn toward the world (and more specifically still, the world of politics). Narratocracy enlists forms of correspondence that designate both the nature of perception and what counts as a subject of perception. As an ethopoetic modality of knowledge committed to justifying the value of appearances, narratocracy thus constitutes us as a specific type of political subject: the literary individual.

Consider, in this regard, Judith Butler's account of the Rodney King video and the verdict in 1992 in the trial of the officers charged with using excessive force in his beating. Her concern stems from an act of perversion: namely, the defense council's successful presentation of the Rodney King beating by the Los Angeles police officers at the scene as a threat to those same officers. "How could this video," she asks in astonishment, "be used as evidence that the body being beaten was *itself* the source of danger?"[36] Her answer, quite rightly, is that the kind of viewing that the jurors were being asked to do took place within "a racially saturated field of visibility."[37] The rendering readable of the Rodney King beating to the jurors involved arranging the visual evidence within what Butler calls "a racist disposition of the visible"[38] that counted the black male body as a signifier for danger to the law.

Butler's reaction and response to the perceptual preconditions for the Rodney King verdict is to enlist "an aggressive counterreading" that reads "not only for the 'event' of violence, but for the racist schema that orchestrates and interprets the event, which splits the violent intention off from the body who wields it and attributes it to the body who receives it."[39] In other words, Butler's solution asks us to change the story line in order to render the Rodney King video differently readable, that is, readable in such a way that the phantasmagoric racial episteme at work during the trial is demystified.

It is hard to disagree with such a conclusion, but I think there is a parallel strategy, beyond the narratocratic one proposed by Butler, that may be pursued. We can recall, as Butler does, that the tactic of visual presentation adopted by the defense council was to slow down the video, break it into staccato sequences, and eliminate the soundtrack. The jurors didn't hear the sexual and racial obscenities shouted by the Los Angeles police officers but only saw punctuated scenes of potential violence. Within a legal system that requires certainty in order to convict, the defense council's objective was to transform the certainty of police violence into the certainty of Rodney King's threat (thus rendering the police violence uncertain): that strategy, in short, enacted a reconfiguration of the sensible that exploited an interruptive sequence of visual stills.

But what if rather than pursuing an aggressive counterreading that shifts the register of symbolic identification to unveil a racial visual field, we pointed out the dynamics of sensation that accompany the techniques of image production? What if the prosecutors in the Rodney King trial had made evident the techniques deployed by the defense council that transformed viewing into reading? That is, what if rather than remaining within the confines of a literary subjectivity where viewing *is* reading, a counterparsing took place that displayed not only the racialized viewing practices of the jurors but also the narratocratic technologies that rendered readable the defense council's reversal of violence?

Focusing on how the slowing down of the video and the elimination of the soundtrack transformed the viewing subject into a reading subject, for instance, might expose the fact that all viewing occurs within a regime of perception that parses what is and is not sensible.[40] Moreover, it could also reveal how the transformation of viewing into reading requires the deployment of specific epistemic technologies that guarantee the available correspondences between perception and meaning. Though an aggressive counterreading may be successful in rearticulating the symbolic structure of identification, the scene of production for that symbolic structure remains the same (i.e., a discursive and deliberative one) as do the conditions of its intelligibility (i.e., viewing as reading).[41] By moving beyond the narratocratic impulse of providing counternarratives, we confront the ethical demands of visuality that reside in the production of the image, or the cropping of the frame, with the hope of disrupting the capture of a racialized conviction.[42]

A modest amendment to Butler's invitation of an aggressive counterreading, then, might turn to Ludwig Wittgenstein's discussion of reading in the *Philosophical Investigations*. "Try this experiment," he writes, "Say the numbers from 1 to 12. Now look at the dial of your watch and read them.—What was it that you called 'reading' in the latter case? That is, what did you do to make it into *reading*?"[43] Those familiar with Wittgenstein's writings will recognize how this passage reiterates the idea of perspicuity that structures his famous duck-rabbit example.[44] What is it about a sequence of stenographic marks, he asks, that renders them readable? Many answers may be given to this question, but one answer, recently proposed by Linda Zerilli, is particularly helpful. In *Feminism and the Abyss of Freedom*, Zerilli explains that Wittgenstein's dawning of an aspect (in our example, the difference between saying numbers and reading a watch dial) presumes that ordinary seeing functions in such a way that "we normally understand without interpreting, and that is not a defect of some kind or failing on our part but the nonreflective basis of anything we might call critique."[45]

The relevance of Zerilli's assertion is twofold: first, that any form of aspect dawning is premised on ordinary seeing, so that we always already exist within the confines of a regime of perception which is not necessarily an illusory or subjectifying mode of existence. Secondly, and more significantly, by drawing a distinction between saying numbers and reading the watch dial, Wittgenstein is asserting that there is nothing in the watch that compels a readerly engagement. To put it in Zerilli's own words, "the dawning of an aspect allows one to see that what one sees is not ascribable to anything in the object, but is rather based on the use of another concept."[46] To say this, in the end, is to insist that our perceptual activities are at once particular and percept driven, and that though we might ordinarily engage with objects in a narratocratic mode, there is nothing in the activity of critical political theorizing that requires individuals to have to accept or submit to narratocracy as the standard by which actions, events, and subjectivities are at once articulated and rendered meaningful.

Though I find Linda Zerilli's project in *Feminism and the Abyss of Freedom* compelling and persuasive,[47] I depart from her analysis at the point when she asserts that "the possibility of interrupting and altering the system of representation in which we decide the question of true and false involves the faculty of presentation or figuration,"[48] that is, the imagination. For Zerilli, the imagination holds the place of Butler's "aggressive counterreading" that, I want to suggest, is an activity of configuration subsequent to the event of interruption. To be sure, I don't disagree with Zerilli that the imagination is a crucial political faculty; nor do I disagree with her claim, implicit in her discussion of aspect dawning, that the imagination might be helpful in enabling an internal feminist critical practice. I do however want to suggest that the possibility of interrupting systems of representation can occur without having to rely on the faculty of the imagination. Or, to put it slightly differently, in this book I argue that the experience of sensation disarticulates received forms of subjectivity and regimes of perception, and that the event of disarticulation precedes the productive role of figuration or presentation that Zerilli attributes to the imagination. I expand on this point, in somewhat different terms, in my discussion of Kantian immediacy in chapter 1. There I argue that Kant is committed to two moments of aesthetic experience: the first is the immediacy of aesthetic impact, and the second is the pronouncement of an aesthetic judgment, after the experience. I see the work of figuration as crucial to the second moment. Whereas in the first instance, when we are captured by a sensation, we do not require the determinative power of the faculty of the imagination to figure the newly thinkable. Indeed, in this moment it is disfiguration that is doing the work of interruption.

In chapter 1 I work out the aesthetic and political dimensions of sensation that will guide me throughout the rest of the book. This chapter, entitled "From *Nomos* to *Nomad*: Kant, Deleuze, and Rancière on Sensation," is the most expository piece of writing in this book, and, as a result, it is least like the others. Whereas the subsequent chapters pivot around particular objects of aesthetic and political attention as sources for theoretical reflection (like a festival, a piazza, a movie, or a morsel of food), this chapter is exegetical in its attempt to offer a reinterpretation of Kantian disinterest informed by the aesthetic and political insights of Gilles Deleuze and Jacques

Rancière. In contrast to those who criticize Kant for his theory of the subject and also in contrast to those who endorse the political relevance of the third critique for its account of communicability, I argue that Kant's aesthetic writings present a theory of the decentered subject and a political critique of privilege in aesthetic reflection. For Kant the "disinterested interest" of aesthetic judgment that arises from the immediate intensity of an aesthetic experience does not describe an impartial judicial stance but refers, rather, to a radical suspension of the subject from any ambition or desire of impartiality. This point, I argue further, forms the backdrop for the aesthetico-political orientation shared by Deleuze and Rancière and in the second half of this chapter, I address the debt that Deleuze and Rancière have to Kant's *Critique of Judgment*.[49] Ultimately, what we have with the triangulation of Kant on immediacy, Deleuze on indistinction, and Rancière on dissensus is an exploration of sensation as a radical democratic moment in aesthetic judgment: rather than taste being inextricably bound to privilege, on Kant's, Deleuze's, and Rancière's account there is no ground for privilege because there are no rules to determine the beautiful and hence, no reliable sources of authority to impose aesthetic standards.

In chapter 2, I expand on this point by shifting emphasis. If narratocracy is a problem for contemporary theory, then a source for this problem is historiographical accounts of political thinking that define political speech as the discovery and development of artifacts called concepts.[50] In "The Piazza, the Edicola, and the Noise of the Utterance," I address these narratocratic biases and argue that those proponents of a history of rhetoric that treat the utterance as if its sole purpose is to present a cognitive claim overlook the sensoriality of claim making and, especially, the aurality of the utterance. In these pages I pursue a subjunctive history of democratic culture and introduce a theory of the utterance attentive to those aural qualities (like sonority and duration) that extend beyond its semantic and grammatical boundaries. Relying on the work of Michel de Certeau, Wassily Kandinsky, and Mikhail Bakhtin, I argue that an attunement to the aurality of democratic culture reconfigures our perceptual appreciation of what political claim making can sound like. In the concluding sections I examine the role of the Italian piazza as a documentary source for the political life of sensation. An attention to such cultural objects composing the diurnal life of a demos like the piazza and the *edicola* (newsstand), I conclude, makes available a democratic form of nonsense that is not absent sense or meaninglessness, but rather refers to practices of articulation that stand outside of the shared lexicon of deliberation.

Much current historiography sets the narratocratic standards for theoretical argument. Through reading and writing, a concept transforms into the material stuff of theory. But such transformations rely on the presupposition of a communal sense that spans the centuries and establishes, beyond any doubt, the relationship between the expression of language, the advancement of a theoretical proposition, and a reader's posture of theoretical attention. The exploration of such presuppositions informs my analysis of Niccolò Machiavelli's writings. In the chapter entitled "Machiavelli's Theory of Sensation and Florence's *Vita Festiva*," I examine the history of public festivals in Renaissance Florence and consider how the explosion of the *vita festiva* (festival life) in the late quattrocento and early cinquecento might have contributed to Machiavelli's own understanding of the *vivere civile* (civic life). In so doing, I argue that in order to appreciate the political culture of the *vita festiva*, we must attend to the multiple plateaus of the political life of sensation crucial to this culture. As important as conceptual clarification may be to ideational artistry, there is another domain at work in Machiavelli's oeuvre that emphasizes the role of indistinction and brings with it an interruption of the regimes of perception and a reconfiguration of our forms of political reflection. This moment, I explain, begins with the impact of the "iter" of iteration and extends to the *riscontro* (clash, or encounter) of sensation.

At the core of my genealogical investigations is the claim that reading and writing are not simply exegetical enterprises but are, importantly, ethopoetic practices. Shifting from historical concerns to more contemporary ones, the subsequent chapter entitled "The Viewing Subject: Caravaggio, Bacon, and *The Ring*" is an engagement with recent studies in visual culture and their possible contributions to contemporary political thought. Here, I discuss a pictorial tradition developed by Caravaggio and expanded by the Irish painter Francis Bacon, both of whose visual efforts exploit the possibility of experiencing an aesthetic object without the imperative of rendering it readable. I pursue this insight in my discussion of the film *The Ring* which, I suggest, portrays practices of viewing so as to make specific claims on the viewer about the viewing experience. I argue further that the insistence of these aesthetic forms on the act of looking rather than on anything resembling a story puts pressure on political theory's own commitment to reading and writing as privileged forms of visual engagement. I conclude that though the citizen subject may have been a reading subject, the contemporary citizen subject is a viewing subject. Contemporary democratic theory, then, would be well served to engage the micropolitical strategies that restrict "viewing" to mere "seeing" and that limit circulation to only one posture of visuality.

The final chapter, entitled "You're Eating Too Fast! Slow Food's Ethos of *Convivium*," asks the following question: is there such a thing as a taste for politics? This chapter begins with an analysis of the mouth as a complex organ of political reflection and the role of flavor as an important thematic consideration in the history of political thought. Included in this genealogy of flavor are the writings of the nineteenth-century gourmand Pellegrino Artusi, whose recipes I discuss in order to set the stage for the ecogastronomic critical interventions of the Slow Food movement against culinary globalization. My interest is to explore Slow Food's ethos of convivium that, I argue, relies on a principle of transversality that is neither utilitarian, rationalist, nor communicative but is, rather, organoleptic: it endorses a *living with* the world that invites an appreciation of how the divergences and dissimilarities of tastes, textures, and flavors appear in the diurnal dimensions of sensory life.

In the concluding epilogue I reprise my considerations of an ethics of appearance in democratic politics (via a discussion of the Abu Ghraib photographs) and focus on a distinction that structures the entirety of this book. Namely, the difference between treating an aesthetic object as an instance of meaningful expression or as an occasion for responsiveness (what I previously referred to as an *attending to* the world). In both instances there is an account of aesthetic experience as crucial to political reflection. At stake in this distinction, however, is the possibility of considering the advent of an appearance as a potential act of part-taking in the ethopoetic practices of the political life of sensation.

CHAPTER ONE

From *Nomos* to *Nomad*

Kant, Deleuze, and Rancière on Sensation

> Thus although critics, as Hume says, are able to reason more plausibly than cooks, they must still share the same fate. For the determining ground of their judgment they are not able to look to the force of demonstrations, but only to the reflection of the subject upon his own state (of pleasure or displeasure), to the exclusion of precepts and rules. IMMANUEL KANT

One of the most challenging political and aesthetic demands posed by the work of Gilles Deleuze is "to have done with judgment."[1] "If it is so disgusting to judge," he affirms, "it is not because everything is of equal value, but on the contrary because what has value can be made or distinguished only by defying judgment."[2] The difficulty with judgment, Deleuze unremittingly argues throughout his oeuvre, is not that it creates distinctions that disable the possibility of equality; the problem, rather, is that in order for something to have value, it must traverse the criteria of judgment that enable the appraisal of value. Value, as Kant also showed in his *Critique of Judgment*, is an intensity that is not produced through judgment or by it but is, instead, that which exceeds any interest there might be in judging. Thus, in order to have value, we must do away with judgment.

To overcome judgment, Deleuze introduces the possibility of indistinction: a condition whereby those regimes of perception that structure one's appraisals are disarticulated and rendered indistinct from one another.[3] Indistinction is Deleuze's way of characterizing an engagement with the world that overcomes the necessity of referentiality and the legislative urge that accompanies a referential model. Drawing sustenance from Melville's famous scrivener, Deleuze explains how Bartleby's formula is "devastating" precisely because it renders the preferable and nonpreferable indistinct;[4] "I would prefer not to" is an antiformalist formula that challenges the insistence of pointing to one's preferences and having those preferences count as the referential coordinates that will constitute a life's trajectory.

In a critical and engaged response, Jacques Rancière addresses his distress regarding Deleuze's work, especially Deleuze's late writings on literature.[5] That distress is, for him, epitomized by one of Deleuze's more unusual images: "a world 'in process, an archipelago', which is that of fraternal individuals: 'A wall of loose, uncemented stones, where every element has a value in itself but also in relation to others'."[6] Rancière's apprehension is guided by what he considers an implicit quietism that accompanies the archipelago image. His ultimate concern is that the motility promised by indistinction is also an indifferentism since indistinction denies the possibility of judgment, and hence also its political potential of critique and disruption. For Rancière, Deleuze's loose surfaces force us to slide up against a brick wall of uncemented stones, no longer allowing us to stand against anything. Indistinction, he worries, comes dangerously close to indifferentism "and the question remains how can one make a difference in the political community with this indifference?"[7]

In this chapter I undertake an exposition of, and engagement with, a Deleuzian disgust with judgment. I do so by bringing Deleuze and Rancière into conversation with one another and by showing the proximity of these thinkers' theoretical articulations. To do this, I establish the Kantian origins of their respective positions on judgment. Specifically, I am interested in how Deleuze's treatment of indistinction and Rancière's treatment of dissensus and the interruption of the partitions of the sensible are indebted to Immanuel Kant's exposition of the durational intensity of immediacy in aesthetic experience and the disinterested interest that arises in an aesthetic encounter.[8] This triangulation of theoretical positions—that is, Kant on immediacy, Deleuze on indistinction, Rancière on dissensus—configures the theoretical trajectory of my own explorations of the political life of sensation throughout this work.

My motivation for this triangulation is equally threefold. The first is theoretical: I argue that the experience of sensation does not rely on a preconstituted composition of individual subjectivity or consciousness. My treatment of Kant, Deleuze, and Rancière will show how these thinkers share an insight about the nature of perception and the composition of common sense. Furthermore, I will show how Deleuze and Rancière, indebted to a Kantian insight about the nature of aesthetic experience, extend that insight and transform it into a critical project that takes issue with the possibility of a perceptual common ground for the distribution of sense.

The second point is an ethical one: the compulsion to legislate judgment and provide a common source of norms for appraisal coincides with an instrumentalist urge to dictate the conditions of possibility for value that are subsequently deployed to direct political action. This second observation regards the relationship between freedom and the experience of value, and my development of it is indebted to Immanuel Kant's claim that in aesthetic experience there can be no rules to legislate a judgment of the beautiful. Though Kant's account of immediacy and disinterest is not original in that it can be situated within a more general, eighteenth-century fascination with the moment of aesthetic impact,[9] what is original is his commitment to resisting any deontological account of the beautiful. Kant believes that our aesthetic judgments cannot be indebted to an authoritative knowledge, nor can they be commanded by it. Rather, an experience of the beautiful is such that it ungrounds our subjectivity and compels a form of reflection that cannot rely on an inherited structure or a preorganization of values.[10]

Finally, my third motivation is an aesthetico-political one: my argument throughout this book is that within any one regime of perception there exists a micropolitics of appraisal that formulates the shared conditions for sense making. These micropolitical strategies create dynamics of conviction that generate affinities of sensibility between and among individuals and groups. More than what has wittingly or unwittingly been endorsed as a "clash of civilizations,"[11] contemporary democratic life is characterized by varying and diverse political cultures of conviction, each of which carries its own regimes of perception that govern what does and does not count as an experience, motivation, or intuition. These regimes of perception constitute a common world of the sensible which, at one and the same time, distributes legitimacy and endorses the convictions that bring that sense world into being. Kant, Deleuze, and Rancière, I argue, are thinkers attuned to the dynamics of interruption and reconfiguration of sense making that the experiences of sensation afford.

Kantian Immediacy

"Those Ideas which are rais'd in the Mind upon the presence of external Objects, and their acting upon our Bodys, are call'd Sensations," asserts Francis Hutcheson. "We find that the Mind in such Cases is passive, and has not Power directly to prevent the Perception or Idea, or to vary it at its Reception, as long as we continue our Bodys in a state fit to be acted upon by the external Object."[12] Hutcheson's definition of sensation insists not so much on the separation of mind and body as on the relative independence of perception from the rational faculties. The passivity of the mind, for Hutcheson, refers to the inertness of the intellectual faculties in determining the event of sensation. As Paul Guyer explains, "Hutcheson does not just argue that the sense of beauty is natural and immediate, but he also excludes from its operation precisely the kind of manifestation of the faculty of reason which is ultimately central to Shaftesbury's Neoplatonism."[13] For Guyer, Hutcheson represents a break with the Neoplatonic commitment to integrating sensorial receptivity with intellectual comprehension that the Earl of Shaftesbury had defended so strongly in his 1711 publication, *Characteristics of*

Men, Manners, Opinions, Times. A subsequent inheritor of Hutcheson's intervention is Immanuel Kant, Guyer explains further, whose treatment of the disinterested interest in the judgment of beauty pays tribute to some of Hutcheson's key insights into the nature and origin of sensation.

Implicit in Hutcheson's argument regarding the radical separation of sensation and the intellect is the assertion that that which is consequent to sensorial perception—aesthetic experience—cannot lay a claim to use or advantage (this includes the use or advantage of an aristocratic posture of aesthetic detachment endorsed by the Earl of Shaftesbury).[14] Since the rational faculties determine the use value of an object and since those faculties are, in principle, inconsequential to aesthetic experience, it follows that the possibility of identifying use value through aesthetic experience is equally unavailable. It is this insight that forms the backdrop to Kant's own reflections on the disinterested interest in aesthetic judgment, as he explains in the first part, section 5 of the *Critique of Judgment*: "Of all these three kinds of delight [i.e., pleasant, beautiful, and good], that of taste in the beautiful may be said to be the one and only disinterested and free delight; for, with it, no interest, whether of sense or reason, extorts approval."[15]

For Kant, there is an important resonance between freedom and disinterest that has nothing to do with a Neoplatonic idealism. Kant's claim is not one that attempts to decontextualize aesthetic experience by insisting on its disinterested nature: that is, Kant's "disinterest" should not be read in the same light or with the same critical purchase as "impartial."[16] It is, instead, exactly the opposite. The disinterested interest in aesthetic experience, which at the end of part 1, section 5 becomes the basis for Kant's definition of a judgment of the beautiful, is the result of a radical suspension of the subject of perception from the conditions that would make the desire for impartiality and ambition worth pursuing. For Kant, the beautiful is a kind of hybrid experience that is neither purely rational (like the good) nor purely sensorial (like the gratification of the pleasant), but is at once both and neither. Beauty belongs to reason to the extent that it concerns human beings, and human beings are rational creatures to the extent that they possess the mental capacity to generate representations; beauty is irrational to the extent that it appeals to our sensory perceptions; but it is neither to the extent that neither reason nor sense dictate the terms of our acknowledgment of beauty. In this regard, neither reason nor sense legislates the possibility of our experience of the beautiful, and thus neither reason nor sense "extorts our approval." Rather than the disinterested subject being a version of the impartial observer, what Kant offers his readers is a subject whose interest at the moment of sensory experience is disarticulated, as are his or her conditions of subjectivity.

The feeling of freedom that arises from aesthetic experience occurs because there is no governing principle in the beautiful that commands a submission to its mode of attention. The disinterested interest in the beautiful is thus a claim about the impossibility of generating a relationship of want between an object and the subject of perception. This lack of interest further extends Hutcheson's original claim that use value is irrelevant to aesthetic experience. For Kant, like Hutcheson, the possibility of establishing the use value of an object requires the further possibility of generating conditions for assigning comparative value to that object vis-à-vis other objects within a series. Thus, we have a relationship of use when we can assess the value of an object in relation to other either similar or dissimilar objects. But in the case of aesthetic judgment, no such relationship can exist. The question remains why.

To answer this question, we must revert to the preceding section of the third critique, section 4 of the first part. This section sets out to explain that the desire for the good carries an interest as does the desire for the pleasant. Because the good belongs to the legislative faculty of reason, Kant explains, and its prescription depends on knowing the nature of that good thing, one must be able to give reasons for the goodness of something as well as to conceive or represent it. Kant's basic point is that a concept of the good needs to be in place in order to direct our actions, and our justifications of the normative conditions that compel us to sign on to a particular conception of the good determine our interest in it. To use a thoroughly conventional Kantian example, we have an interest in not lying because we would not want to be lied to. But the beautiful, Kant emphasizes repeatedly, is exempt from this dynamic of a necessary relation between object and subjective interest.

To stress the point, there is a difference here that marks the nature of the disinterested interest in the beautiful: that difference, I want to argue, is a durational one. By the end of the subsequent paragraph, after instructing his readers on the distinction between the pleasant and the good, Kant makes the following passing remark:

> But that the reference to delight is wholly different where what gratifies is at the same time called good, is evident from the fact that with the good the question always is whether it is mediately or immediately good, i.e., useful or good in itself; whereas with the agreeable this point can never arise, since the word always means what pleases immediately—and it is just the same with what I call beautiful.[17]

Kant never expands fully on this last clause, nor does he explain why the word "agreeable" always signifies immediacy. We are left to deduce, therefore, that the immediacy of which Kant speaks must have something to do with the manner in which an external object impacts upon our senses and the reverberations generated subsequent to that immediate impact. The beautiful shares with the pleasant the condition of sensation, and thus also shares the durational intensity of immediacy. Immediacy in aesthetic experience, I submit, interrupts the capture of interest and makes it so that there can be a disinterested interest in the beautiful.

This can occur for two reasons: first, under the pressures of immediacy we lose access to the kinds of conditions that make it possible to determine things like motivation, use, or belief—all forces that constitute the nature of interest. Second, in such a temporal condition we lack the necessary cognitive connections to generate comparisons. When we encounter an aesthetic object, Kant believes, that object has an immediate impact on our senses, thus generating sensations. The immediacy of that impact is a durational intensity that interrupts the circuitry of interactivity to which we are accustomed. That is, with the immediacy of sensory perception, we cannot rely on any structure that would relate that object to other sources of value because at that moment our capacity to create lines of connection (like analogy or comparison) is interrupted. In short, we lack the opportunity of generating a regime of value necessary to establish a context of interest that would relate an object to other objects. It follows from this that when an aesthetic object captures us, the encounter with that object disarticulates the purchase of belief we deem necessary for conviction. Here, conviction occurs through the durational intensity of sensation, and not from an a priori interest; from a Kantian perspective, the capture of conviction cannot result from an antecedent methodological or interpretive commitment or belief.

To claim an interest we must also be able to connect an object with a set of other objects and subsume that object under a general category that organizes its comparative value. This, in effect, is the basis of any utilitarian value scheme to the extent that, by creating a representational device for collecting members of a group in a common activity (like a dean's honor list, for instance), one is able to generate an appraisal of their relative standing vis-à-vis other members of the same group (i.e., the student's ranking).[18] The immediacy of aesthetic experience, however, interrupts this operation, ushering us into a state of judicial convalescence; all of a sudden, we cannot determine the category to which that object belongs nor are we equipped to determine its place in any serial disposition of other objects. Thus, there is a "disinterested interest" in a judgment of the beautiful because we have a natural disposition to aesthetic experiences (to the extent that we are creatures of sensation, and thus equipped to react to an object); but when we do encounter an aesthetic object, we at once lose the capacity to relate that object to any conventional or customary regime of value. The durational intensity of immediacy in aesthetic experience interrupts the posture of attention that has interest as its guiding objective; or, to put this in terms that will become more familiar to the reader as we proceed, immediacy disrupts an interest-oriented regime of appraisal, and with it, it disfigures the organoleptic conditions for signification. In short, aesthetic experience ungrounds our subjectivity.

When Kant famously defines taste as "the faculty of estimating an object or a mode of representation by means of a delight or aversion apart from any interest,"[19] he is referring to the moment of immediacy that denies any antecedent conceptualization of the beautiful object. Kantian aesthetic judgment thus attends to a disjunctive moment when we are unable to make the kinds of distinctions necessary to establish an interest in an object, including any antecedent relation like tradition, context, or function. Indeed, Kant's commitment to disinterest goes so far as to assert that we must be indifferent to the existence of the object,[20] and though Kant readily admits that we exist within a substratum of sensorial affinities that organize our world according to determinable partitions of perception, and that such partitions themselves are organized according to norms and practices of sense making, aesthetic experience is such that it interrupts those networks of relation by creating a temporal and temporary state of indistinction.

It's worth pointing out that there is nothing in Kant's claims about immediacy that make it synonymous with quickness or speed. Immediacy is a durational intensity that refers to the moment of impact as well as to the protracted state of attention of the subject engaged with a beautiful object, what Kant will refer to as our tendency to "dwell [or linger] on the contemplation of the beautiful."[21] In this regard, we can assume that part of what constitutes the pleasure of aesthetic experience for Kant results from the condition of capture and conviction that comes from the immediacy of an aesthetic encounter. And the reason why we might conclude this is that, given its temporal nature, the possibility of such encounters are unprescribable, and hence impossible to legislate.[22] In other words, the pleasure in the beautiful (that stems from the immediacy of a disinterested interest) is the result of the sensation of freedom subsequent to an encounter with an object without the burden of having to attend to a conceptual framework that defines or justifies the nature of one's conviction. There is a pleasure for Kant in not being bound by concepts, as he clearly states: "To deem something good, I must always know what sort of a thing the object is intended to be, i.e., I must have a concept of it. That is not necessary to enable me to see beauty in a thing."[23]

The formidableness of this assertion is made manifest in what I will refer to throughout this book as Kant's radical democratic project in the *Critique of Judgment*. I have partly hinted at this by including an epigraph that aligns critics and cooks, a passage that places their judgments of taste on an equal footing. But though Kant was clearly amused by this passage in Hume's essays—or at least amused enough to treat it at length—he also takes this principle very seriously. When Kant speaks of a "principle of taste," he refers to the possibility of subsuming the value of an object under a general rubric that will guide the acceptance of its beauty. To do so, however, would immediately disqualify the object's claim to beauty. "Thus," he concludes, "*there can be no rule to which anyone is to be compelled to recognize anything as beautiful.*"[24] I will return to this assertion in my discussion of the transversal properties of an ethos of convivium in chapter 5. For now, I want to connect this claim both to the temporality of immediacy and to the notion of a disinterested interest.

Kant repeats versions of this claim throughout the third critique. Most notably, he introduces the language of the a priori in section 12 of the first part to assert the impossibility of determining a priori grounds for legitimating the feeling of either pleasure or pain. Once again, as in the case of immediacy, the justification is temporal: one cannot know a priori whether something will be pleasant or painful because pleasure and pain are consequent to experience, and hence are a posteriori phenomena. More precisely, there can be no interest in the existence of the beautiful object because there also cannot be any possibility of determining a concept for it. That is, the disinterested interest in the beautiful trumps any and all motivation for legislating an object's worth. Moreover, and as already indicated, the immediacy of the moment of aesthetic impact will also deny the possibility of a rule governing the beautiful for if immediacy interrupts our regimes of perception to the point of discomposing our way of attending to the world, we must conclude that that immediacy will also disrupt our relationship to rule and rule following.[25] Just as we cannot establish an interest in a beautiful object that will continue through time and regardless of the spectator, so it will be impossible to establish a rule for the preservation and prescription of beauty. To put the matter slightly differently, immediacy and disinterest make it impossible to determine rules for aesthetic reflection.[26]

This antinormative thread that runs throughout the third critique is what I take to be Kant's radical democratic project of aesthetic judgment. His description of the feeling of freedom that comes with a relief from the burdens of normativity is indicative of this, but so is his collapsing of the rank status between the cook and the critic. As I argue, the account of aesthetic experience that is grounded in the durational intensity of immediacy and a disinterested interest in the existence of the object works to coordinate the conditions that make possible this radically egalitarian position. For Kant, anyone can experience beauty precisely because no one can determine its conditions of existence. This is the egalitarian promise of Kantian aesthetics: both the cook and the critic are afforded the occasion for aesthetic experience and neither the cook nor the critic has the privilege of safeguarding the conditions for that experience. Taste is available, for Kant, regardless of privilege.

That there "can be no rule to which anyone is to be compelled to recognize anything as beautiful" is Kant's most endearing performative contradiction, but it is also Kant's most impressive expression of the relationship between freedom, equality, and aesthetic judgment. It is, I would argue further, a moment in the political life of sensation when the regimes of appraisal with which we customarily organize the world are taken from us, compelling us to have to reconfigure our own postures of attention. Through aesthetic judgment, then, we are subject to the whim of a moment that is unlike any other moment; and the consequence of this indeterminate technique of subjectification is the disarticulation of the conventions by which we attend to the world.

Deleuze's Disgust with Judgment Examined

What seems profoundly perplexing about Deleuze's disgust with judgment is the extent to which his aversion is indebted to Kantian judgment despite his resistance to it.[27] As we have just seen, immediacy and disinterest work in such a way as to create precisely the conditions of indistinction that are, for Deleuze, at once aesthetically and ethically crucial for the kind of descendental ethics of sensation he develops. Before I describe the nature of that ethical project, I want to outline what is at stake in Deleuze's appeal "to have done with judgment."[28]

We get a sense of those stakes when Deleuze claims that the doctrine of judgment, elaborated from Greek tragedy to modern philosophy, is characterized by the institution of the tribunal. "Kant," he goes on to say, "did not invent a true critique of judgment; on the contrary, what the book of this title established was a fantastic subjective tribunal." The tribunal, he then expands, is "that infinite point at which accusation, deliberation, and verdict converge."[29] Judgment for Deleuze is inseparable from a Kafkian image of a trial where the pronouncements of a judge are dangerous liaisons that direct the referent to the referee and the arbiter to the *arbitrium*. The "fantastic subjective tribunal" that Kant establishes refers to a kind of submission the individual goes through in the process of reflection, not unlike the Christian examination of conscience in confession;[30] and it is this process of submission that Deleuze finds most disgusting. Indeed, by insisting on disgust as the manner by which we might engage the doctrine of judgment qua model of tribunal, Deleuze is in fact deploying a principle he will sustain throughout his aesthetic and ethical writings: "The doctrine of judgment has reversed and replaced the system of affects,"[31] and his project will be to invert that reversal.

To do so, Deleuze explores the possibility of an ontology of sensation.[32] By this, I mean that Deleuze's critique of the doctrine of judgment insists on the nondeterminable, affective dimensions of human life. In this respect, Rancière is absolutely correct when he describes Deleuze's project as substituting "one ground for another, an empiricist English ground for a German idealist ground."[33] The "empiricist English ground" is the system of affects that Deleuze derives from his studies of David Hume and that he wants put in the place of the "German idealist ground" of the Kantian tribunal.[34] But there is something more to Deleuze's admonitions against judgment than this significant reversal; Deleuze's commitment to an ontology of sensation is rooted in an attempt to grapple with the relationship between thinking and sensation without having to revert to a synthesis of mind and body which, for him, is implied by, and constitutive of, the judgment model. Thus, the basis of Deleuze's refusal of Kantian judgment rests on a belief that the work done to provide a real theory of imaginative freedom is ultimately curtailed by the Königsbergian's desire to synthesize the cognitive and the experiential; that is, by his profound need to make freedom palpable. It is, ultimately, this process of synthesis—and the subsumptive operation that enables it—which allows Deleuze to equate Kantian judgment with the image of the tribunal.

Deleuze's critique of the model of judgment thus has two parts: (1) judgment involves the operation of subsumption of the particular to the general which implies the legislative authority of the general in organizing the distribution of particulars, and (2) in order for this operation to occur, there must be presuppositions in place that constitute a sensible regime of the common that establishes the channels for the distribution of things, the reception of those things by specific subjects, and the ends to which those things ought to be disposed.[35] In other words, the model of judgment can never escape the forces of legislation and distribution, and subsumption is the cognitive operation that enables the fluid working of these forces. Thus, Deleuze concludes, "judgment has precisely two essential functions, and only two: distribution, which it ensures by the *partition* of concepts; and hierarchization, which it ensures by the *measuring* of subjects. To the former corresponds the faculty of judgment known as common sense, to the latter the faculty known as good sense (or first sense). Both constitute just measure or 'justice' as a value of judgment."[36]

The "fantastic subjective tribunal" of Kant's third critique is Deleuze's judgment of Kant and refers to Kant's failure in establishing what he sets out to do: namely, to create conditions of judgment that do not rely on a normative regime of interest. This objection might be easily dismissed given my exposition of Kantian immediacy in the preceding pages, and though Deleuze might sign on to my initial analysis, Kant's failure, he might retort, is not in his account of aesthetic experience per se but with his account of the consequences of this moment within the larger framework of his critical philosophy. Kant's failure, in other words, stems from the kind of universality that he reserves for the judgment of the beautiful. For Kant, when we say that something is beautiful, we assume that it is valid for everyone even though we cannot legislate it to be so. This is the principle of universality that forms the basis of his discussion of the *sensus communis*. This expectation of communicability, Deleuze wants to say, is what reestablishes the tribunal regime of appraisal that is the model of judgment. Here is one of Kant's formulations of the *sensus communis*:

> However, by the name *sensus communis* is to be understood the idea of a public sense, i.e., a critical faculty which in its reflective act takes account (a priori) of the mode of representation of everyone else, in order, as it were, to weigh its judgment with the collective reason of mankind, and thereby avoid the illusion arising from subjective and personal conditions which could readily be taken for objective, an illusion that would exert a prejudicial influence upon its judgment. This is accomplished by weighing the judgment, not so much with actual, as rather with the merely possible, judgments of others, and by putting ourselves in the position of everyone else, as the result of a mere abstraction from the limitations which contingently affect our own estimate. This, in turn, is effected by so far as possible letting go the element of matter, i.e., sensation, in our general state of representative activity, and confining attention to the formal peculiarities of our representation or general state of representative activity.[37]

Much has been said about this famous passage, and I will refrain from further commenting on it other than to point out that when Kant speaks of the communicability of a judgment of taste, he is no longer talking about the immediacy of aesthetic experience. On the contrary, the discussion of *sensus communis* answers the question of how to circulate and transmit one's experiences so as to avoid the potential of coercion; that is, the emergence of a public sense refers to what occurs subsequent to aesthetic experience. In this regard, everything about this passage returns us to a utilitarian framework: Kant's fear that one's subjective judgment could transform itself into a coercive and authoritarian injunction (i.e., "a prejudicial influence") is so strong that the intersubjectivity implicit in the idea of a "collective reason of mankind" becomes the instrumental objective of aesthetic experience. Moreover, once Kant establishes the condition of universality that "is effected by so far as possible letting go the element of matter, i.e., sensation, in our general state of representative activity," he also establishes the conditions for analogy that, in the second part of the third critique, ground his claim that "the Beautiful is the symbol of the morally Good, and that it is only in this respect (a reference which is natural to every man and which every man postulates in others as a duty) that it gives pleasure with a claim for the agreement of everyone else."[38]

The mistake that Kant makes, in Deleuze's view, is that though he is willing to allow the possibility of an experience that does not require the conditions of legislation to enable it, he ultimately does not allow that experience to disarticulate the system of hierarchy that would determine it. Rather than giving us a theory of the freedom of the imagination from the determination of concepts, Deleuze concludes that Kant's final critique "uncovers a deeper free and indeterminate accord of the faculties as the condition of the possibility of every determinate relationship."[39] That the beautiful is a symbol of the morally good means, for Deleuze, that the morally good has instrumental priority over the effects of the beautiful. In other words, though we enter into a condition of indistinction in aesthetic experience, that condition does not interrupt the hierarchy of the system of value that forms the basis of a Kantian critical philosophy. Once Kant invents a symbolic relation between the moral and the aesthetic, he establishes a rank order of value that ultimately privileges and immunizes the moral domain. Thus, whereas from one perspective Kant's synthesis of the moral and the beautiful (that completes his synthesis of the transcendental and the empirical) may appear as a commitment to the idea that our sense of beauty is complicit with a myriad of other sources of human value,[40] from Deleuze's perspective the symbolic relation between the moral and the aesthetic is both the first and last phase of a tribunal that establishes the privilege of the moral in a doctrine of the faculties.

What is more, an analogical relation such as the one established through a symbolic accord between the moral and the aesthetic returns us to the problem of distribution because it endorses a system of identity; analogy is, for Deleuze, "the essence of judgment"[41] to the extent that it determines a system of distributive value relations where "existence is cut into lots, the affects are distributed into lots, and then related to higher forms."[42] When Deleuze thus concludes, in *Kant's Critical Philosophy*, that "the last Critique uncovers a deeper free and indeterminate accord of the faculties as the condition of the possibility of every determinate relationship," he is in fact condemning Kant for having succumbed to the determinative power of analogy, and for having reinstituted a regime of appraisal that curtails sensation from doing the work of disfiguration that Kant himself had promised in his account of aesthetic experience. By introducing analogy as a relevant category in his analysis, Kant simultaneously reintroduces the determinative powers of subsumption and subordination as apodictic principles for the organization of experience.

For Deleuze, analogy is a privileged form of judgment that is synonymous with subordination; through analogy we make things similar, and thus subsume the particularity of an experience to a general rule or category. Through the determinative power of analogy one is compelled to have to measure up to preestablished conditions of representation. Judgment is thus a rigid designator for subordination, and even the greatest attempt to escape this dynamic, Kant's *Critique of Judgment*, was ultimately unsuccessful.

Deleuze's Reply: A Descendental Ethics

Where Kant retains a principle of hierarchy that determines the primacy of moral reasoning through the subordination of the beautiful to the moral, Deleuze proposes a *descendental* ethics that engages the aesthetico-political dynamics of subsumption and subordination at the *infraficial* level of experience. To be subordinate means to belong to an order below or beneath someone or something; "to subsume" is the verb that accounts for the dynamic of subordination. Subsumption and subordination operate in such a way as to create strata under which the intensities of sensation are assigned. In this respect, there is an infraficial plateau generated at every moment of judgment. If judgment corresponds to subsumption, then each instant of judgment figures a surface under which an intensity is fixed; the line that draws this boundary traces a stratum which is the infraficial plateau. Deleuze's descendental ethics engages and interrupts the line's capacity to figure such infraficial surfaces and in doing so attempts to expose the intensity of sensation.

Consider, in this regard, Deleuze's discussion with Félix Guattari of the line's relationship to writing:

> In effect, the line is all the more abstract when writing is absent, either because it has yet to develop or only exists outside or alongside. When writing takes charge of abstraction, as it does in empires, the line, already downgraded, necessarily tends to become concrete, even figurative. Children forget how to draw. But in the absence of writing, or when peoples have no need for a writing system of their own because theirs is borrowed from more or less nearby empires (as was the case for the nomads), the line is necessarily abstract; it is necessarily invested with all the power of abstraction, which finds no other outlet.[43]

Writing is characteristic of empires, in Deleuze's and Guattari's often difficult account of these entities because writing is an activity for the figurative display of comparative value: a word's meaning is constituted by its position within a context of possible significations, including the context of a sentence—that is, the organizational structure of the sentence is such that it puts pressure onto individual words to perform their role.[44] The written line is not abstract because writing always has a context; thus, as Antoine de Saint-Exupéry famously recounted, once taught the adult skill of writing, children forget how to draw.[45] Writing is here understood as a technique of figuration that gives shape to things and halts the movement and migration of words. Reminiscent of the distinction between an outline and a contour invoked by Merleau-Ponty in his discussion of Cézanne's apples (see the prologue), the aesthetic distinction between abstraction and figuration marks the possibility of thinking ethics in terms other than nomological ones.

It is important to note that for Deleuze and Guattari the oscillations between abstraction and figuration are not specific to any particular historical period but rather are characteristic of a nomological turn that accompanies the desire to subordinate the line to the figure. As Daniel Smith explains, "the danger of figuration or representation is that it is both illustrative and narrative: it relates the image to an object that it supposedly illustrates, thereby subordinating the eye to the model of recognition and losing the immediacy of the sensation."[46] This, I would add, is also the danger of nomology, and it is this dynamic—that is, the passage from the abstract to the figurative that subordinates sensations to the nomological imperative of "making sense"—that is the central concern of a Deleuzian descendental ethics of indistinction. "The figurative, or imitation or representation," Deleuze and Guattari continue,

> is a consequence, a result of certain characteristics of the line when it assumes a given form. We must therefore define those characteristics first. Take a system in which transversals are subordinated to diagonals, diagonals to horizontals and verticals, horizontals and verticals to points (even when there [*sic*] are virtual). A system of this kind, which is rectilinear or unilinear regardless of the number of lines, expresses the formal conditions under which a space is striated and the line describes a contour. Such a line is inherently, formally, representative in itself, even if it does not represent anything. On the other hand, *a line that delimits nothing, that describes no contour*, that no longer goes from one point to another but instead passes between points, that is always declining from the horizontal and the vertical and deviating from the diagonal, that is constantly changing direction, a mutant line of this kind that is without outside or inside, form or background, beginning or end and that is alive as a continuous variation—such a line is truly an abstract line, and describes a smooth space. It is not inexpressive. Yet is true [*sic*] that it does not constitute a stable and symmetrical *form of expression* grounded in a resonance of points and a conjunction of lines. It is nevertheless accompanied by *material traits of expression*, the effects of which multiply step by step.[47]

The system of subordinations that creates a hierarchy ranging from the transversal line to points is characteristic of the nomological which has as its guiding principles the representative power of figuration and narration.[48] The purpose of that system is to establish a regime of perception where the line is exclusively representative, describing a contour rather than allowing the contour to resonate as Merleau-Ponty had said it might. In short, nomology's power is to represent through figuration or narration. In contrast, the abstract line has the intensity of Bartleby's "I would prefer not to;" it declines narration, figuration, and the need to describe referentiality. Such a line is not inexpressive but is, rather, a sensation "accompanied by material traits of expression." These material traits of expression are the systems of affects that resonate along the infraficial plateau of indistinct sensation.

The aesthetico-political claims about abstraction and figuration vis-à-vis the nature of a line are emblematic of an entire thematic running throughout Deleuze's oeuvre: that is, the movement from *nomos* to *nomad* involves a descent into the infraficial domain of sensation. Subsumption, subordination, and the like are intensities of figuration that gain purchase once the system of representations and subordination is put into place. But at their generative stages, before they emerge and acquire a nomology about them, these intensities persist on a plane beneath the surface, and at this infraficial plateau, there is nothing about them that guarantees their nomological purchase. This, ultimately, is the moment of indistinction that Deleuze's entire oeuvre wants to keep alive.

Indistinction thus refers to an inability of figuring, of giving an account that is something other than an acknowledgment of sensation. In this regard, indistinction also refers to the transversalism of a descendental ethics that aspires to the state of judicial convalescence Kant described in his account of aesthetic experience, that is, when our postures of attention are disfigured to the point of no longer being subject to the perceptual conditions determined by a regime of perception. At that moment the dynamics of conviction that capture our attention are disarticulated and our comfortable repose of figuration is, in a word, disfigured. The political shift from nomos to nomad has an accompanying aesthetic shift from sense to sensation (i.e., from figuration to disfiguration), and it is the engagement with the dynamics of this shift that best characterizes Deleuze's descendental ethics.

This moment, I argue, is cognate with Kant's moment of immediacy. Just as Kant believes that there can be no rules for judging beauty because there is no determining ground at the moment of aesthetic encounter, so does Deleuze believe that the moment of indistinction is immediate and precedes the generic and qualitative (one might even say "figural") account of difference. The indistinction of sensation is Deleuze's corollary to a Kantian disinterested interest: in both cases, immediacy works to create a condition of dissensual delight where we can no longer be confident of any determinate relation between perception and organoleptic experience. Indeed, Deleuze takes it one step further to the extent that he imagines each moment of experience as a potential moment of disfiguration, which helps explain his fascination with the Irish painter, Francis Bacon. Bacon, as we shall see in chapter 4, is the painter of disfiguration who refused the narratological necessity of justifying the scream; he is, to put it in more linear terms, someone who explored the line's potential beyond (or beneath) its figural qualities. This aesthetic resistance to figuration is, finally, what structures Deleuze's descendental ethics.

Jacques Rancière's Dissensus

Deleuze's indistinction presents an argument about equality: "The world of representation," he asserts, "presupposes a certain type of sedentary distribution, which divides or shares out that which is distributed in order to give 'each' their fixed shares."[49] The problem with such systems of distribution (and with representation more generally) is that they can never adequately account for those heterological elements whose particularity does not fit. The apportioning of parts relies on an arrangement whose organizational structure must remain intact in order for the operation of partitioning to take place. Indistinction is the aesthetico-political intervention into that world of common parts and common distribution channels. If, that is, the channels of distribution of equality become indistinct (including our networks of perception), then we have no way of assigning a privileged participation to any one experience or criterion of experience.

If there is anything that Gilles Deleuze and Jacques Rancière share, it is this distrust of the criteria of distribution that rely on predetermined lines of communication, of "counting" as Rancière might say. "A surface," Rancière explains, "is not merely a geometric composition of lines. It is a certain distribution of the sensible."[50] By this he means that those spaces we recognize as properly political spaces, surfaces upon which political action takes place, are subject to what I have been calling a regime of perception, where our modes of perceiving and the micropolitical strategies that direct our perceptive attentions determine the nature, shape, and form an appearance can take. What is more, these dynamics also determine our modes of attending to phenomena: in the case of reading and writing, to continue with the example discussed above, our eyes follow the words from left to right on a page (moving from the top left-hand side to the bottom right, in the case of most North Atlantic pagination typecasts and word processing programs): this is a distribution of perception along a surface made up of a geometric composition of lines. And this regime of perception, with its distributions and assignments of attention, has repercussions for what we consider a legitimate mode of sense making. A distribution of the sensible addresses the modes of attending to the world that align our organoleptic practices with our bodily postures, our cognitive attunements, and our practices of sense making. Thus, the partition or division of the sensible (*partage du sensible*) is "the cutting up [*decoupage*] of the perceptual world that anticipates, through its sensible evidence, the distribution of shares and social parties. And this distribution itself presupposes a cutting up of what is visible and what is not, of what can be heard and what cannot, of what is noise and what is speech."[51]

The apportioning of perception creates geometric outlines that establish a surface upon which value might fluidly circulate. This, in the end, is the basis of Rancière's category of "the police" at the heart of his critique of Althusser.[52] Contradicting the claim of interpellation, he explains how Althusser's petty officer is not an agent of interruption, as the account of recognition through interpellation might suggest. Rather, the main ambition of the police is to increase the flow of circulation, to move traffic along when the traffic lights don't work, if you will. Rancière's "there is nothing to see here" of the police order contravenes Althusser's "Hey, you there!" by showing us that the work of the police (and what Deleuze and Guattari will also call the work of "the organization of the organs of the organism"[53]) is to ensure the proper circulation of things within a system so as not to leave unaccounted the supplemental elements whose value has, as of yet, been unassigned. A distribution of the sensible is at one and the same time a modality for the assignation of value, or a criterion of judgment.

Dissensus, then, is Rancière's synonym for politics: it is not the opposition or disagreement of interests between established groups in any dynamic system but rather is "the production, within a determined, sensible world, of a given that is heterogeneous to it."[54] Dissensus thus refers to the emergence of a heterology extraneous to a common world of perceiving and, through that emergence, a disruption of the mechanisms that enable the fluidity of the operation. Dissensus is an interruption that disarticulates the distributions of perception that enabled its own emergence. In this regard, Rancière concludes, "politics is aesthetic in that it makes visible what had been excluded from the perceptual field, and in that it makes audible what used to be inaudible."[55] That is, dissensus is an aesthetico-political moment that results in the reconfiguration of the regimes of perception that seize our attention, so that we can no longer assume the legislative authority (or logical priority) of any one form of perception.

For this reason it becomes impossible to equate Rancière's claims about visibility and audibility with a politics of recognition. That is, it's not at all the case that dissensus makes it so that we recognize noise as speech, or recognize a particular group as counting as part of a larger genus; rather, dissensus refers to the ways in which the dynamics of recognition delimit the possibilities of visibility and sayability. Recognition, in this regard, would fall under the auspices of the police order's organization of circulation; or, as Deleuze might say, recognition requires analogy to the extent that it requires a "methodological continuity in the perception of resemblances."[56] This is because a politics of recognition presupposes that there is always an order in place that may be recognized and that can count as a standard of audibility and visibility. Dissensus, on the other hand, disrupts the perceptual continuities required to endorse recognition; it not only reconfigures the field of appearance of politics but also—and crucially—the processes of perceptual subjectification by which individual and collective human bodies constitute themselves as appearances.

The problem with Deleuze's indistinction, Rancière thus explains in thoroughly Deleuzian terms, is its implicit atomism: "no other fraternity is normally formed, only atoms and groups of atoms, accidents and their incessant modifications."[57] The atomistic nature of indistinction, in other words, takes from us the power to organize. Whereas Rancière imagines dissensus as comprising both the power of disfiguration and reconfiguration of the perceptual world—and thus, ceteris paribus, the power to act as the political supplement to a regime of resemblances that is always already exclusive—he does not imagine in Deleuze a similar possibility of reconfiguration. In short, Rancière does not see in Deleuze a strong account of relationality, and if it is true that Deleuze substitutes the British empiricists for the German idealists, his disgust with judgment is so intense that it undervalues the play of relationality so prevalent in eighteenth-century accounts of sensation.

There is a sense in which Rancière's accusation of atomism is excessive: Deleuze does have a rich account of relationality both in his discussion of the threefold nature of repetition and, in his work with Guattari, on the forces of territorialization and assemblage. But there is also a sense in which Rancière's claim is equally accurate. Deleuze's indistinction is taken with Kant's idea of immediacy, and immediacy is an account of aesthetic experience that is radically individuating: it isolates the figures of experience and by isolating them, disarticulates them. It describes, in short, a state of stupor that dismembers the common grounds for referring to the world. But though this moment accurately describes Deleuze's account of indistinction and its Kantian origins, it is no less an accurate account of Rancière's dissensus: dissensus refers precisely to that aesthetico-political moment of heterogeneity Kant described in his *Critique of Judgment*. The disinterested interest one experiences in a judgment of the beautiful is the result of an interruption of the networks of distribution that grant us a common ground. Disinterest, disfiguration, and dissensus are the names given to this experience of sensation.

The claim I defend in this chapter is that Deleuze's and Rancière's aesthetico-political reflections carry an indebtedness to a radical democratic moment in Kant's *Critique of Judgment*. I describe that moment, as Kant does, in terms of his antinormative account of aesthetic experience resulting from the durational intensity of immediacy, and the disinterested interest consequent to the moment of capture in an aesthetic encounter. In the following chapters I keep in play the triangulation of this theoretical moment elaborated by Kant, Deleuze, and Rancière, as well as the aesthetic, political, and ethical tensions such a triangulation engenders.

CHAPTER TWO

The Piazza, the *Edicola*, and the Noise of the Utterance

As to why I appear today in this unaccustomed garb, you shall now hear, if only you will not begrudge lending your ears to my discourse—not those ears, to be sure, which you carry to sermons, but those for which you are accustomed to prick up for mountebanks in the marketplace, for clowns and jesters, the ears which, in the old days, our friend Midas inclined to the god Pan. DESIDERIUS ERASMUS

From the clamor of voices overrunning and breaking up the field of statements comes a mumble that escapes the control of speakers and that violates the supposed division between speaking individuals. MICHEL DE CERTEAU

In March 2000, thousands of chocolatiers took to the piazzas of Italy to showcase their chocolate. It was an odd scene because it could easily have been confused with one of many commercial endeavors. In this case, however, the public preparation of chocolate was meant as a protest against new standards instituted by the European Chocolate Directive on March 15, 2000. The European Commission wanted to alter the composition of chocolate, something many independent continental European chocolatiers couldn't swallow. The Directive had rebaptized chocolate; it stated that any form of chocolate with 5 percent vegetable fat could be called chocolate despite the fact that most European chocolatiers made chocolate primarily out of cocoa and cocoa butter. The introduction of vegetable fats as a substitute for cocoa butter—as in the case of most mass-produced, chocolate-flavored snacks—would not only significantly alter the economy of developing regions (an estimated loss of about 800 million dollars in Africa and South America, the largest producers of cocoa in the world)[1] but would also force people to alter their sense of what counted and tasted like chocolate. Not to mention the fact that this would cause the price of cocoa to increase, they argued, making "pre-Directive chocolate" a luxury item. So the chocolatiers occupied the piazzas with their pots, pans, and camping stoves, creating an impromptu chocolate taste test to, as it were, "prove their point."

What can be said of such forms of civil unrest? Can the preparation of pre-Directive chocolate in the piazzas of Italy be considered a political utterance? If so, what kind of utterance is it and how are we to attend to it? The problem with addressing such forms of political expression, it seems, lies in the fact that our tools of political reflection are contoured by a narratocratic model of communication based exclusively on semantic exchange. But is a political utterance—what we still recognize as the basis of deliberation, communication, and the right to free speech—reducible to the shape of the sign or is there something in an utterance that extends beyond its stenographic outline?

With broad strokes I will address some of these questions by broaching the possibility of an aural history of democratic culture. But why? Why should the aurality of an utterance matter to an inquiry into the political life of sensation? One possible answer lies in the fact that democratic cultures are noisy and disorderly things, that the institution and functioning of democratic structures of government differ dramatically from the cacophony of democratic politics and that in order to better grasp the intentions, hopes, and motivations of emerging democratic movements, we need to be attuned not only to what people want but to the regimes of perception that govern our postures of attention. Indeed, the problematic link between democracy and noise was established early on in the history of political thought. In the *Republic* (554a) Plato complains about those barbaric noises imported from Italy that inaugurate a "theatrocracy," a rule of the spectacle. "The noise of number—the very custom of applauding, imported from Italy—is what has created theatrocracy," Jacques Rancière explains. "Power is not so much in the spectacle itself as in the racket that it authorizes."[2]

The growing tendency to export democratic principles of government to regions where these are said to be absent presumes that human needs and wants not only are the same throughout the world but, more importantly, that they are expressed and understood in the same manner regardless of geography, faith, or language. Simply put, democracy is viewed exclusively as a set of principles of government that, like the grammar of a language, can be delineated, taught, and applied so that when uttered, it will sound the same regardless of habits of reading or listening. This trend towards a grammatical and linguistic common sense also finds expression in theoretical debates about normativity and deontology in contemporary liberalism. These debates reduce our appreciation of political utterances to the shape of the moral claim, making it the most reasonable mode for the exchange of political value.

But there is a second factor at work here: the adoption of an ideational approach to language when studying the cultural life of a polity. Over the past several decades cultural and political theorists, ethicists, and historians alike have developed a rich program of study for the analysis of the concepts that configure our political imaginaries. Much of this research is indebted to the principles of linguistic analysis outlined by Ferdinand de Saussure in his *Course in General Linguistics*. But a cursory reexamination of Saussure's writings points to a fundamental inattention of the ideational approach: the conceptual top-heaviness of the linguistic turn's approach to the study of democratic deliberation (whether at the level of speech-act theory, communicative action, or normative proceduralism) has sacrificed the flip side of the Janus-faced coin of Saussurian linguistics, namely the phoneme or sound-image that sources our sensory impressions.[3] In other words, debates in democratic deliberation about signification (i.e., the signified) subsume the equally important role of the linguistic signifier, or the noise of the utterance.

"Unaware of our typographic cultural bias," explains Marshall McLuhan, "our I.Q. testers assume that uniform and continuous habits are a sign of intelligence, thus eliminating the ear man and the tactile man."[4] Such Gutenbergian assumptions, I contend, result in a de facto partition between those who can and cannot speak, between appropriate and inappropriate verbal sounds, between those who have the authority of the word and those whose speech is unofficial. With such divisions in place, modes of expression like the baking of pure chocolate are treated as mere blabber or worse, as cultural extravagances. But given the cacophony of democratic life it seems worthwhile to ask ourselves whether only one mode of address should be given normative priority in political communication. That is, could it not be the case that when we treat the noise of an utterance as babble something politically relevant is lost? It may be that when we utter something that isn't semantically significant (by which I mean either meaningful or useful) it is nonetheless valuable because it compels us to have to reconfigure the requisite conditions for perceptual attention.[5]

In what follows, I propose an account of the utterance attentive to those qualities that extend beyond its semantic texture and grammatical boundaries. Democratic politics, I suggest, is first and foremost a politics of noise. Though a political utterance may be retroactively tuned to sound like a reasonable expression of interests, its first pitch is an interruptive noise. In this respect, I want to know what such dissensus sounds like: what is the noise of the utterance?

I begin by looking at the utterance as a tool of historiographical analysis. Theorized as an instance of meaningful communication, the utterance grounds a history of conceptual exchange that situates the terms of political discourse within a context of a reasonable language which is the history of political thought. The precariousness of this history rests on the foundational idea that, when speaking, individuals are saying something and that it is the task of the historian as the raconteur of the "what was said" to explicate the meaning of these statements. Relying on the ocular caress of the historian's eye who resuscitates a discourse of the dead, we realize that political speech is meaningful speech. The result, as Michael Warner explains, is that "the poetic or textual qualities of an utterance are disregarded in favor of sense."[6] And, I will add, so are its vocal and aural qualities.

After exploring the possibility of an aural history of the utterance, I shift my attention to the Italian piazza. The piazza is a source of evidentiary support for the noise of the utterance. Relying on its architecture and role in popular culture, I suggest that the piazza creates a spatio-temporal plateau of diverse forms of perceptual part-taking. What occurs in the piazza is never simply reducible to what can be seen, read, or argued. Rather, the piazza is a space where disjunctive vectors of movement create enunciative possibilities that extend well beyond the perceptual correspondences of the narratocratic. I conclude by discussing a recent cultural heritage renovation project of a nineteenth-century *edicola* (newsstand) in Piazza Garibaldi, Casalmaggiore—a small, northern Italian town on the Po River bordering Lombardy and Emilia Romagna.

A History in the Subjunctive

A word is sound and sense. There is no neutral voice, explains Roland Barthes when speaking of the grain of the voice.[7] The same can be said of the historical text: the written word has a "grain" that our reading habits, reduced to the silence of the eyes hovering over the page, overlook. Roger Chartier argues that "reading is not uniquely an abstract operation of the intellect: it brings the body into play."[8] Indeed, the distinction between the literate and the illiterate worlds, the high and low cultures of history, is insufficient to understand the aural qualities of the reading operation. Recall Carlo Ginzburg's Menocchio, a figure whose literary competencies were limited and unsanctioned but who nonetheless was able to create an entire cosmology that challenged the Friuli religious authorities of his day to the point of enlisting inquisitorial persecution.[9]

The scholar interested in the utterance as a departure point of political thought must consider the varieties of readers, their communities and habits of reading, but also the possibility that what we understand today by reading has not always been the same kind of operation. No text exists independent of its physical support, and, despite the literary and hermeneutic ideal of a text whose meaning is sustained notwithstanding the differences in forms of expression or material apparatus, the book remains a material object. It does not simply contain words that constitute meaning but, as a physical object, it interacts with the body in ways that go well beyond the ocular scan. Using only our sight to visualize the meaning of a historical utterance is to censor ourselves and those whom we read to only one reading habit: namely, our own.

John Locke, attuned to the nuances of the materiality of the text, reminds us of the nauseous effects of introducing duration—that is, a "breathing space"—into sacred literature: by breaking up the Bible with headings, paragraphs, and numbered passages, one divides the word of God, he argued.[10] As a consequence, every sect and anybody who could read would be able to use scripture to justify their own insights and legitimate their beliefs. What Johns Rawls called the "historical origin of political liberalism"[11] is, according to Locke, the result of a somatic reconfiguration of the materiality of the reading page that makes God's words available to anyone living in a post-Gutenberg galaxy.

The materiality of the book is one place, among many, where we may begin an investigation into the noise of the utterance. What Chartier calls "the silent production that is the activity of reading" is both the problem and the condition of our current understandings of democratic deliberation. What exists outside of this "silent production" becomes—almost automatically—relegated to the domain of the unintelligible, thus creating one of the most extreme forms of presentism in contemporary historiography. "History," explains Jacques Rancière, "can become a science only through a poetic detour . . . It doesn't give this to itself in the form of an explicit philosophical thesis, but in the very texture of narrative, in the modes of interpretation, but also in the style of the sentence, the tense and person of the verb, the plays of the literary and the figurative."[12] The spoken utterance, whose sense is unavailable to literary forms of representation, is thus no literary text at all; it cannot receive proper theoretical attention because its conditions of legibility and intelligibility can only be surmised. Hence, the noise of the utterance—the tone, pitch, and sound that the murmurings of a people could be imagined to make—must belong to a conjectural history of unintelligibility that remains at once without documents and undocumented.

"Such is history," states Michel de Certeau:

> A play of life and death is sought in the calm telling of a tale, in the resurgence and denial of the origin, the unfolding of a dead past and result of a permanent practice. It reiterates, under another rule, the myths built upon a murder of an originary death and fashions out of language the forever-remnant trace of a beginning that is as impossible to recover as to forget.[13]

The interstitial space where the dead word is brought to life through the tranquil narrativizing operation of the historian is also the locus of that which cannot have a place in history. Through the writing of history, de Certeau tells us, the past is made present not only because it is retold but because it is told through the viewing of the historian who reads the past in the same manner and with the same purpose as one reading in the present. The operation of writing a past omits what was said and heard because the noise of the utterance cannot be read. The writing of history is a credentialing institution that "forms the collection of documents [by] exil[ing] them from practice in order to confer onto them the status of abstract objects of knowledge."[14]

Carlo Ginzburg notes that the culture of popular classes is largely oral but, as we have just surmised, any historical analysis that attends to the at once oral and aural elements of a culture might be subject to suspicion, or regarded simply as conjectural. Thus, we are warned, we must pay attention to written documents because only these can provide us with an accurate taxonomy of the past. But this approach seems undemocratic. Attending only to the written word to ground a history of democratic culture disrespects the "residue of unintelligibility"[15] in those clamorous elements that resist typographic specificity. Moreover, we must admit that the kind of tact that comes with an appreciation of the moderated word, bound by the stenographic margins of the written page, or illustrated by the familiar linguist's diagram of two heads exchanging meaning, is not a democratic quality at all: Tact, as Nancy Struever's work on Renaissance rhetoric shows, is "an essential ingredient of courtliness"[16] and thus an aristocratic virtue of restraint that has little to do with the tumults of democratic insurrection.[17] Indeed, the tactful word involves the kind of discipline that one finds in Castiglione's *Book of the Courtier*—a handbook of courtliness that stands in sharp contrast to, say, Machiavelli's defense of republican tumults in the *Discorsi*.[18]

The anchoring of a past through the narrativization of archival documentation is, I submit, a problem for histories of political thought interested in democratic culture. What such histories require is a shift in historiographical mood. Rather than being expository, the recounting of noise invokes the subjunctive: an aural history of democratic culture is a history in the subjunctive; it is a genealogy of political reflection attentive to, as Erasmus extols, the pricking of the ears.

The Clamor of Voices

Democracies are noisy creatures born of what Hannah Arendt refers to as the "unquiet" (*askholia*) of the *vita activa*.[19] There are no adequate testimonies to this noise; yet, we can assume that democracy and noise go hand in hand. I imagine that there has never been a quiet democratic movement, like there has never been a peaceful democratic uprising. "Political interlocution," Jacques Rancière tells us, "has always mixed up language games and rules of expression. . . . The problem," he continues, "is not for people speaking 'different languages,' literally or figuratively, to understand each other, any more than it is for 'linguistic breakdowns' to be overcome by the invention of new languages. The problem is knowing whether the subjects who count in the interlocution 'are' or 'are not,' whether they are speaking or just making noise."[20] The Esperanto fantasy of a common language for deliberation is unveiled when we realize that, at every moment when there is an interruption in the logic of "rule," deliberation is advanced not by an unreasonable comprehensive doctrine but by the utterances made by those whose language is not common. In popular literature, the distinction between speaking and making noise differentiates the adult from the infant; likewise, as Rancière suggests, such a distinction differentiates semantics from mere blabber, from those who have the authority of the word, and those who are "just making noise."

To better explain this distinction, it is worthwhile to consider the founding metaphor that grounds many accounts of deliberation in contemporary democratic theory: the literary economy of meaningful exchange. Rooted in an ideal of a barter economy, this founding trope requires a balanced distribution of (in this case "semantic") goods resulting in common understanding between speaking subjects. Thus, despite the often misinvoked Wittgensteinian metaphor of "the language game" intended to explain the procedural aspects of deliberation, what gets overlooked is the notion of unproductive loss implicit in the practice of games.

The loss of energy expended in participating in a competition, however, has no end other than the game itself. Consider the huge sums of money spent on the salaries of baseball players or on staging presidential debates. Consider also the money spent on the construction of stadiums, training, maintenance, and (in our day) sponsorship: the *telos* is the intangible pleasure derived from the consumption by the spectator (either through watching the game, participating in betting, or purchasing products endorsed by the stars of the game). Yet such pleasure is pure loss since once the game is finished, all that is left is a used and expired ticket. To be sure, I am not suggesting that sporting events are not worthwhile. But I am suggesting that within the contours of the logic of a barter economy, they are entirely useless. And yet, they are nonetheless crucial to the functioning of a well-ordered society. Georges Bataille calls this element of pure loss "nonproductive expenditure" and finds exemplary expression for it in such forms of primitive exchange as *potlatch* and in such institutions as games (gambling, athletics, etc.), cults and religions (through sacrifice), and art (his example is poetry).[21]

This element is neglected in descriptions of democratic deliberation that concentrate on the narratocratic production of meaning and overlook the nonproductive expenditure of noise. Intersubjective exchange of the kind described by theorists and historians of narratocracy eschews the element of play in language games by grounding communication in a barter economy where the energy expended must, in the last resort, always be productive (i.e., "meaningful"). Simply put, the connotation of a "balanced account" (or consensus) that grounds the deliberative scenario is intended to assuage the fear of "not wasting one's breath" when talking. Such an imperative sacrifices noise as an active element in communication because, after all, noise is nothing other than wasted breath.

Consider, in this regard, the following: "To understand any serious utterance," Quentin Skinner tells us, "we need to grasp not merely the meaning of what is said, but at the same time the intended force with which the utterance is issued. We need to grasp what people are saying but also what they are doing in saying it."[22] Skinner's classic formulation is the methodological basis for much work in the history of ideas. Skinner began his groundbreaking studies defending the core notion that "the concept of truth is irrelevant to the enterprise of explaining beliefs."[23] In so doing, he forwarded a procedure for the analysis of historical texts based on the Austinian distinction between an utterance's meaning and its illocutionary force. To gather the illocutionary force of an author's statement, Skinner argued, we must first and foremost gather an understanding of the context within which the utterance is made: whom is the author addressing in writing and to whom is she responding? So, it is not simply the meaning of the sentence that matters—the "what was said"—but also the "what was meant in saying what was said."

Importantly, this differs from the truth of the intended meaning of the author, as if it were possible to get inside an historical author's head, as it were, from the documents she or he left behind. Skinner distinguishes sharply between the philosophical meaning of a statement and its intended meaning; in this respect, he argues, we cannot stop at the meaning of the statement itself and assume that our rules of interpretation—whether grammatical, philosophical, linguistic, and so forth—are universally valid. Rather, what we need to do as historians of ideas—the office occupied by anyone who reads historical texts—is to get at the stakes involved in making those statements, and for this we need to be able to appreciate the historical context within which the author is writing.

The crucial corollary to Skinner's argument is, by now, a familiar one: the performative aspect of an utterance—what an author was doing in saying—is accompanied by the equally important realization that "any act of communication will always constitute the taking up of some determinate position in relation to some pre-existing conversation or argument."[24] Thus the history of ideas which Skinner defends is a history of "moves in an argument;"[25] it is a history of rhetoric that imagines that what an author is doing in making utterances is arguing and that in doing so, she or he is expressing her or his beliefs. Skinner's key contribution, with the introduction of an Austinian philosophy of language into the methodological debates in historiography, is to reconfigure our perception of historical statements, moving us from the idea that statements express a linguistic truth to the idea that they express an author's belief. The best we can do as readers of texts is to get at what a statement means by arriving at an understanding of the author's beliefs.

Thus, Skinner argues, historians must abandon the worship of the "incontrovertible fact:"[26] the task of the historian is not the elucidation of truth, it is the demarcation of an ideology that makes the author's statements comprehensible. "The aim," he asserts, "is to use our ancestors' utterances as a guide to the identification of their beliefs."[27] The primary task of the historian, he continues, "must be that of trying to recover a very precise context of presuppositions and other beliefs, a context that serves to exhibit the utterance in which we are interested as one that was rational for that particular agent, in those particular circumstances, to have held to be true."[28] The ability to decipher coherence and to establish a narrative thread of argumentative continuity is the key literary competency a historian must possess when reading historical authors. This not only provides an accurate account of meaning, it also legitimizes the historian's own reading and, indeed, writing operation.

The "serious utterance"[29] is thus the cultural object of historical analysis. For an utterance to count as "serious" it must be consistent with other utterances the author makes because if the author "displays no concern for consistency, if they employ no recognizable modes of inference, we shall have no means of marking off which of their utterances are to be classed as instances of the speech acts of stating or affirming or defending their beliefs."[30] The "law of noncontradiction"[31] becomes Skinner's standard for designating the difference between a serious and a frivolous utterance. If an author's statements don't seem to make sense, Skinner continues, we need to rethink our own reading strategy and assume that we have either misunderstood or mistranslated the series of propositions we are considering.[32] In short, the task of a history of ideas must be to collect and classify "serious utterances," to confer upon these the status of objects of knowledge so as to create a totalizing taxonomy of possible beliefs. The historian's eyes have an editorial function that enable the hand's narrativizing gesture: With "the gesture of setting aside"[33] the serious from the frivolous utterance, political theory can begin.

There is much to praise in Skinner's approach to studying the history of political thought, and I am indebted to his insights. There are, however, also limitations: though Skinner defends the importance of beliefs over truths in the study of history, his desire to privilege the "serious utterance" betrays a commitment to "true beliefs." In other words, Skinner's "more historically minded approach to the history of ideas"[34] that wants to situate historical texts in their intellectual context in order to make sense of what the author was doing substitutes for the concept of truth the concept of a "true belief." A belief might be different from a historical truth because beliefs look to what an author might have considered possible given the ideological context of his or her time. That being said, the objective of the historian is to make those beliefs available to his or her readers and to give those beliefs a textual reference (or linguistic context) that anchors their indisputable accuracy. That accuracy is further confirmed by a narratocratic procedure that gives coherence to an author's beliefs through the law of noncontradiction that, in turn, establishes a consistency between the context of a body of work and its historical emergence. This process transforms a mere belief into a "true belief," and the conclusiveness of a true belief becomes the objective—the emplotment process—of the historiographical operation according to Skinner. Thus, though it may be true that "the concept of truth is irrelevant to the enterprise of explaining beliefs,"[35] for Skinner the concept of a "true belief" certainly is not irrelevant, and the difference between a true belief and a false one is the difference between a serious and a frivolous utterance: that is, the difference is one between making sense by not contradicting oneself and being senseless, between saying something and simply making noise.

The idea that there is a commonsense language that determines the perceptual conditions for the distinction between a true and false belief (by relying on universal standards like the law of noncontradiction) risks falling prey to precisely the same kind of astute criticism that Skinner poses to those committed to studying "historical truths." Moreover, that "comprehension" is the objective of the study of history is not as obvious as Skinner makes it out to be; "comprehension" is an aesthetic value that carries with it a commitment to narrative continuity, mimesis, and the hermeneutic hope that all expression is meaningful expression.[36] Perhaps a point of departure that would help extend Skinner's appreciation of historical context while resisting his commitment to the "serious utterance" might ask if all utterances or speech acts must be examined through a narratocratic proceduralism where the examiner's obligation (both moral and methodological) is to comprehend the utterance. Can the noise of the utterance suggest something other than a claim's meaning? Mikhail Bakhtin and Wassily Kandinsky might help us in answering some of these questions.

From Point and Line to Utterance

"The sentence," Wassily Kandinsky tells us, "is silence."[37] The sentence not only ends with a point (i.e., the period) but as a complete unit of linguistic analysis, it is said to have and make a point as well; it is, within Kandinsky's taxonomy, the linguistic corollary to the figurative point in art. Its colors are blue, its texture is hard, it stands in stark contrast to the geometric line that is, in its turn, an invisible thing whose track is made by the moving point.[38] As sources of motility, Kandinsky's paintings rely on the figural line to compel movement: "[the line] is created by movement specifically through the destruction of the intense, self-contained repose of the point. There the leap out of the static into the dynamic occurs."[39] The difference between a point and a line is the duration introduced by movement; the dynamic leap of the line made by the moving point infuses temporality into something that would otherwise remain still.

It should be noted that Kandinsky's distinction between "point" and "line" echoes Saussure's original division of the sign as "concept" and "sound-image." Recall how in the *Course in General Linguistics*, while detailing the general principles of linguistics in the opening pages of part one, Saussure specifies the dualist structure of the sign and, before ever giving this duality its semiotic names, explains how the linguistic sign unites "not a thing and a name but a concept and a sound-image."[40] The linguistic sign, then, is a "two-sided psychological entity" that has at once a cognitive *and* material component: it is an arbitrary relationship between idea and sound, and "the two elements are intimately united and each recalls the other."[41] A few paragraphs later, Saussure rebaptizes the sign's component features as signified (i.e., concept) and signifier (i.e., sound-image) and concludes his introductory remarks by establishing the temporal quality of the signifier: "the signifier, being auditory, is unfolded solely in time from which it gets the following characteristics: (a) it represents a span, and (b) the span is measurable in a single dimension; it is a line."[42]

The importance of point and line are as evident in Kandinsky's paintings as they are in Saussurean linguistics. As we saw with Skinner's "serious utterance," the argumentative point is also important to a history of ideas. But by relying on a deliberative norm like the law of noncontradiction as a standard for punctuality, the noise of the utterance is transformed into the silence of the sentence, thus losing its temporal and dynamic qualities. Yet, like Kandinsky and Saussure before him, it is worthwhile to recall the simultaneity of the signifier and signified in the creation of the sign, however arbitrary that simultaneity might be: there is a tension between a concept and sound-image that parallels the tensions between a point and a line—and that tension is born of the signifier's duration.[43]

"The utterance," asserts Mikhail Bakhtin, "is an exceptionally important node of problems."[44] For Bakhtin, there is a problem with the graphic representations of communicative exchange found in linguistic manuals: it creates a fictitious image of communication as unified speech flow invested in the relationship between speaker and listener. Such an image attributes a passive role to the listener such that "the active role of the other in the process of speech communication is thus reduced to a minimum."[45] In contrast Bakhtin shifts his attention away from this kind of linguistic formalism and toward modes of responsiveness: that is, he shifts from a spatial metaphor where language possesses a horizon of meaning to a temporal one that focuses on the durational intensity of the utterance.

In contrast to the reductive tendency of treating the entire utterance as if it were only a signified, Bakhtin looks to an actively responsive attitude that transforms the relationship between listener and speaker: always at the cusp of responsiveness, the listener attends to the meaning of what is said but also, and crucially, to the pauses and interruptions in the breathing space of exchange. These pauses indicate the duration of an utterance; they are "the boundaries of each concrete utterance [and] as a unit of speech communication [they] are determined by a change of speaking subjects, that is, a change of speakers."[46] He continues, "This change of speaking subjects, which creates clear-cut boundaries of the utterance, varies in nature and acquires different forms in the heterogeneous spheres of human activity and life, depending on the functions of language and on the conditions and situations of communication."[47] The silence of the period does not determine the beginning or end of the utterance; rather, it is the sound of breath-pauses between the noise of the words that renders completion to an utterance. Recalling Kandinsky, we can say that the utterance has no point. This, of course, does not mean that it is meaningless; rather, meaning is a result of a retroactive, reconfiguring operation that has little to do with the creation of an utterance per se. Or, to put the matter as Bakhtin does, "a sentence, having become an entire utterance, acquires a special semantic fullness of value" that, on its own, as an instance of language or as a grammatical unit, it does not possess. Semantics has a role to play in communication, but its role is a posteriori to the creation of the utterance. Hence the possibility of an utterance being as long as a novel or as short as a "yes" or "no" reply: its duration is determined by the pauses between the noises, not by its comprehensiveness as a semantic unit. For Bakhtin there is no communication, only co-respondence.

In order to work, this account of the utterance requires a reorientation of our postures of attention and our grammatical mood of analysis. Our appreciation of an other's speech requires the subjunctive. Consider, in this regard, the tentative nature of Bakhtin's account: we "guess" the genre of the utterance, we "predict" its duration, we "foresee" its end, we "have a sense of the speech whole which is only later differentiated during the speech process."[48] Such hesitations are not the result of Bakhtin's own imprecision but are the result of a cultural form of expression whose precision is linked to its durational contours rather than its graphic outline. Certainty comes in knowing that the utterance is imprecise because it is not framed by the unit of semantic exchange—by the point of what is being communicated, or the meaningful kernel of knowledge—but by the change of speaking subjects. And this comes after the fact, after responsiveness occurs.

Like the line, the utterance is noise moving through space: a line of flight or a sound wave, if you will. It exists because of the shift in speaking subjects, and its duration is as varied as the number of possible hearers and listeners. Because it is premised on our ability to intuit its completion, its fullness can be felt only through its incompleteness; indeed, what seems like the end of one utterance and the beginning of another might, to someone else, count as an interruption of a unified speech flow. The point is that Bakhtin's theory of the utterance allows for the possibility of interruption to count as a significant element in communication precisely because it is not considered a mistaken moment of exchange; interruption, rather, marks the shift in speaking subjects, the duration of the utterance. In other words, rather than merely rude, base, or tactless (though it can be all these things too, as Bakhtin's studies on Rabelais show), interruption is a condition of responsiveness. The moment when one reader interrupts her reading to ponder what she read, for instance, is as valid as any other moment, and the same holds true for the speaking scenario: the moment when one responds to a speaking subject is as valid as any other, though it may inevitably appear as a tactless intrusion from the perspective of one who does not attend to the noise of the utterance.

Republics of Noise

Democratic persons are noisy creatures. The word "person"—derived from the Latin *per sonare* (meaning to make sound)—refers to an actor's mask which had "a broad opening at the place of the mouth through which the individual undisguised word of the actor could sound."[49] The culture of democratic iteration thus begins with a kind of *trompe l'oreille*, with a making of a noise that may sound familiar but whose cacophony denies the possibility of familiarity. Indeed, the voice of the other—which is the noise of democracy—always sounds senseless.[50]

The senselessness of which I speak, however, is not synonymous with an absence of intention or meaning, nor is it reducible to unintelligibility.[51] Rather, it refers to a field of iteration that operates on registers other than the ones available for sense making. There is, then, a category of speech—a speech genre, if you will—identifiable as democratic non-sense (or babble); such a category does not refer to the content of that speech but rather to its status within the lexicon of a common language of deliberation. The *trompe l'oreille* of democratic non-sense refers to the unauthorized words of those who speak but whose account is unaccounted for.[52] Thus we must not confuse the "non" of non-sense with unintelligibility or meaninglessness. Or rather, we can confuse it as such only when listening to it from a position of authorized discourse. The non-sense of democratic noise is neither empty nor meaningless; it possesses a semantic fullness that, as Michel de Certeau explains, "introduces schism and dissent into the harmony between sound and sense."[53]

The fiction of a common language of deliberation, like the fiction of a common sense that moderates disagreement, appears after the noise of the utterance has moved through the public space of iteration. The supposed harmony between sound and sense is what we must overlook in order to appreciate the noise of the utterance. Such noise counts as an instance of what Michel de Certeau calls *glossolalia*: a form of speech that, like the Bakhtinian utterance, is responsive and "where the possibility of speaking is deployed for itself."[54] Here meaning is anticipated while duration does the work of anticipation: "Glossolalia postulates that somewhere there is speech, [whereas] interpretation supposes that somewhere there must be meaning."[55]

Theorists of democratic deliberation treat speech like the Freudian analyst does the unconscious: "we know that there is something meaningful there," they assert with obstinacy, "and your inability to generate meaning only proves the point further because when speaking, meaning is either present or hidden in the crepuscules of the not knowing how to say something." By championing the cause of liberating meaning from the depths of insignification, such appeals derive a competency to institute meaningful speech from "their capacity to organize a checkerboard of positions that at once authorizes and limits verbal circulation, divides and controls it."[56] But the decomposition of speech into babble, the repetition of elementary sounds that combine syllables and consonants, creates a space of interlocution that stands outside a preordained topos of signification.

The relationship between speech and dominion is an old one. The term "babble" originates with the tower of Babel, the building of which is the second major biblical episode of hubris after the Fall. Genesis 11:1–10 tells the story of a people who settled in a plain in Babylonia, learned how to make fire-hardened bricks, and used them to create "a tower whose top may reach unto heaven; and let us make us a name, lest we be scattered abroad upon the face of the whole earth."[57] Afraid that this "one people" with "one language" would usurp God's rule, God came down from heaven and bestowed upon them multiple languages to create division and confusion. Hence the term "Babel" or "Babylon" from the Hebrew word meaning "mixed up."[58]

This is a short story that takes up all of ten sentences in the Bible, but its relevance is not to be overlooked. The point of the story is that division is the just punishment for the hubris of a people desiring of *arche* [rule].[59] Indeed, the Babel story is a second fall that further disperses the work of naming done by Adam. The fiction of unity that organizes all the species in the world because they were named by the one created by the word of God (logos, spirit, breath) is dissolved by the fiction of dispersal that results from a desire to establish a human *arche* that challenges the rule of God.[60] Meaning literally "to babble,"[61] "glossolalia" recalls this fictional moment of a divided unity resulting from a challenge to an absolute *arche*. At once, babble recalls that second fall: it is the noise of a people who seek their own form of rule.

Relevant for my immediate purposes is the architecture of this scene of division. In the Babel story there is a tower, there is an open space designated as a "plain in Babylonia," there are a people, and there is division brought about by a multiplicity of discordant utterances. This, in short, is the architectural layout of the Italian piazza:[62] there is a central clock tower, an open, directionless space, and a multiplicity of utterances in an equally varied number of dialects. This architectural document—which, to be sure, differs in material form from a stenographic one—is a palimpsest of footsteps and voices where an ethopoesis of space incessantly recalls the organoleptic interruption that fissured the symbolic organization of *arche* in Genesis.

The piazza marks a space but not a place.[63] It has a name but lacks an address. The difference is a notable one. The piazza does not direct movement, although within the piazza there are trajectories and vectors of body and sound motility. The piazza is "composed of intersections of mobile elements:"[64] it can be at once a market, a theatre, a political rally, a coffee house. Unlike the striations of a patterned grid, it does not impose a distribution of bodies. Nonetheless it is a "punto di ritrovo" (literally: "point of rediscovery"), where one rediscovers old and new friends alike. Walking through a populated Italian piazza, at any moment one finds groups of people gathered variously throughout. Each group is a "compagnia," a company in the sense of "someone with whom you keep company." From these groupings, rivalries rooted in divergences from everything from the political to the athletic to the familial emerge.

The most famous festival recalling such rivalries is the Palio in Siena: at once a pageant and an equestrian competition, it claims a history that dates back to the thirteenth century and takes place twice a year, on July 2nd and August 16th, in Siena's "Piazza del Campo." Each neighborhood in Siena, called a *contrada*, is represented in the Palio and is designated by specific vestments, colors, and flags worn by the residents and jockeys. The primary rule of the Palio is that the riders must ride without a saddle, and though it doesn't matter if the rider does not make it across the finish line, it does matter that the horse cross. The Palio thus becomes a kind of republican tribunal that plays out the tensions of competing neighborhoods. Though today's Palio might be purely a folkloric spectacle, it still recalls the paradox of the piazza: it is a space that, though lacking direction and unity, creates a surface of disjunctive liaisons between differentiable elements.

Emerging in Italy in the thirteenth century, the piazza was created specifically to generate and amplify a *senso civico* (civic sense).[65] Its ideal was the Roman Forum that was, throughout the centuries, reproposed in every town as either the piazza of the cathedral, the civic piazza, or the marketplace piazza. "In that sinuous, open-air interior that is the Roman Forum," explains Mario Isnenghi, "one would enter what seemed like a safe space, surrounded by columns and temple walls, in order to be a citizen and devout person, to converse and engage in commerce, to encounter others and be seen."[66] More than just an architectural innovation, Isnenghi explains further, "the piazza is an empty space" that collects its identity from the colors, shapes, structures, and occupants that inhabit it; it is a space that occasions the coincidence of "form and event, permanence and contingency."[67]

The architecture of the piazza plays host to certain structures that repeat themselves. The most obvious of these is the clock tower whose role it is to set the rhythms of the day for those working outside the immediate walls of the city or, indeed, within the neighborhood where the tower reigns. The tower not only self-consciously recalls the tower of Babel,[68] the striking of its bells also set the somatic habits of a people: they signal when to eat, sleep, wake, pray, and so forth. Being the center of much folklore, these structures become characters of popular urban myths; like the bell tower of Santa Maria Maggiore in Rome, famous for setting Rome's other clocks because it is geographically closest to the meridian of another church, Santa Maria Degli Angeli (built in 1702). Before the firing of a cannon became the standard for setting Rome's clocks, each tower's time was slightly different the farther one moved from Santa Maria Maggiore as each clock tower would set itself to the sounds of its closest neighbor. Setting a kind of premodern Greenwich mean time, the clock tower of Rome's Santa Maria Maggiore held the power of both earthly and divine time.

The struggle to possess time is also played out by the competition between piazzas within towns. Isnenghi correctly notes the trinity of the political, religious, and marketplace piazza in every Italian city. The piazza of town hall has its bell tower that is always set differently from the duomo's bell tower. Here, the tension between mundane power and heavenly power is played out on an hourly basis, and the aural resonances tell an Augustinian story of competition between earthly death and eternal life, temporal finitude and divine eternity.[69]

It wasn't until the period between the eighth and ninth centuries that church towers became resonant with bells. This innovation derived from the belief that the noise of a bell would warn away evil spirits.[70] To this day, bell towers ring in the piazzas of Italy when storms (traditionally considered manifestations of the devil) are on the horizon, and the *campanaro*—the one entrusted to ring the bells—protects the town from evil spirits. Thus, between designating time and protecting from evil, the bell tower creates a "spatio-temporal aggregate"[71] of sanctuary that speaks to the diurnal and mundane culture of the piazza. But the bell tower not only resonates outward through the sound waves of the bells, it also casts its shadow onto the surface of the piazza; it is, in itself, a meridian that designates a spatio-temporal arch where bodies appear. The trajectory traced by the sundial-like shadow of the tower is an empty space of "game and commerce, of work and leisure, of official rule and popular power, of conflict and memory."[72]

Within the many spectacles that play themselves out upon the surface of the piazza is also the spectacle of death. At the edge of each piazza there are posted obituaries of the recently deceased townsfolk. Here, people come to pay their respects, dispute the sources of the death, and remember those who have passed on. The piazza, however, is also where the condemned come to die. Piazzale Loreto in downtown Milano is a case in point. In terms of piazzas, Loreto is not attractive for its architecture, but it is an important node of major roads that connect downtown Milano and the massive Centrale train station to the rest of the city and its periphery. At the end of the Second World War, Piazzale Loreto played host to two major scenes of execution: the first, (between August 10, 1944 and April 28, 1945), witnessed the martyrdom of fifteen antifascist Partigiani. Once Milano was liberated, the piazza was renamed the Piazza dei XV Martiri (Piazza of Fifteen Martyrs), and though the name never stuck, the plaque indicating the event survives.

The second great execution in Piazzale Loreto was on Sunday, April 29, 1945. At three o'clock in the morning, the truck carrying the carcasses of the dead Fascist leaders arrived. Among the bodies of the dead were those of Mussolini and his mistress who, having been hung in effigy before, compounded this day's surreal display of grotesque theatricality.[73] Indeed, the theatricality of the exposition of the dead is underscored by the fact that these bodies were hung upside down, extending the classic images of inversion of highs and lows characteristic of popular festive forms.[74] Here we have an exaggeration of grotesque realism not only theorized by Bakhtin but, in fact, intended by the Resistance with the added distinction that, in this liminal scene of life, death, and carnival, each passerby was permitted to inflict on the cadavers whatever form of posthumous punishment they wished. The ire of the people who came to express their sentiments to the dead is encased in an aura of vindication for the betrayal committed by Mussolini's regime. It is not simply a scene of vengeance, but a scene of transgression that purported to be restitution for the country's dead in the war. Word of mouth testimony remembers this day where one woman arrived on the scene, pulled out a gun from her purse, and shot Mussolini's carcass four times; not to be outdone, another elderly lady who, remembering the loss of her son during the war, whipped the Duce's body while uttering the word "*porcun*" (meaning "pig" in Milanese dialect) under her breath.[75]

Gruesome though this scene may be, it is exemplary of the kind of role that the piazza plays in Italian popular culture: to wit, everything occurs in the piazza, from the most tranquil of meetings, sharing a cup of coffee or an *aperitivo* before supper, to the most violent events that display life and death, festival and tragedy.

The piazza is the center of Italian civic life—political, commercial, religious—and it is the source of the utterances (the mother's "porcun") whose noises resonate along with those of the bell tower, the pitter-patter of footsteps, and so forth. Here the sounds that emerge may be forms of argument, but they are also forms of expression that have very little to do with a deliberative model of communication. These are popular sounds that exist and resonate before they can be classified and documented. They can be febrile sounds because barely audible, as well as futile because as intangible as the breath used to utter them. These sounds, however, manage to play a crucial role in public life regardless of their apparent lack of sense.

Piazza Garibaldi, Casalmaggiore

I want to end my reflections on the Italian piazza by discussing one piazza in particular: Piazza Garibaldi in Casalmaggiore, Italy. Founded in the first century CE, as a Roman outpost (*Castra Major*), Casalmaggiore is located on the shore of the Po River in the Padania agricultural region. It is equidistant to Parma, Cremona, Mantua, and Reggio Emilia. It is, in short, a border town on the shores of the river that divides the two northern regions of Lombardy and Emilia Romagna.

Piazza Garibaldi is notable among the thousands of other piazzas in Italy because of recent renovation work done to its *edicola*, or newsstand.[76] The edicola's role in the popular culture of the piazza is relatively recent (first installed in 1899) and due to the massive increases in

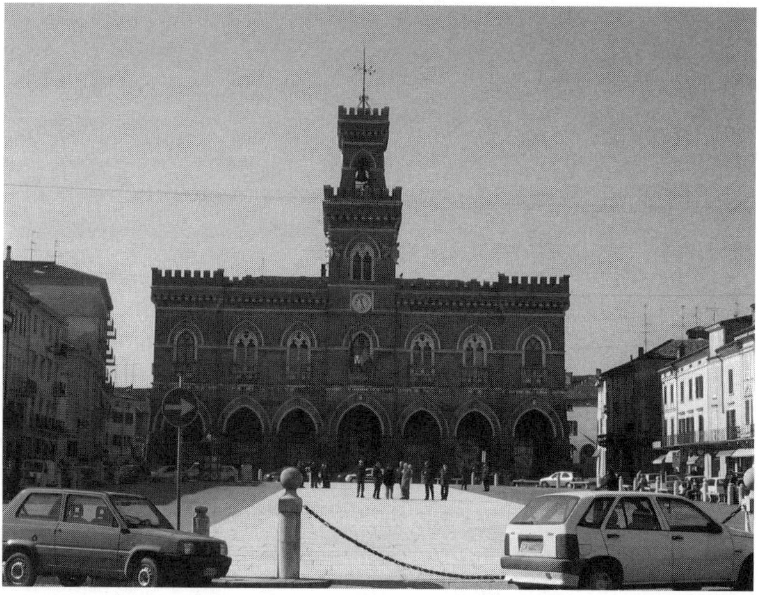

1 "Compagnie" gathering in Piazza Garibaldi, Casalmaggiore, Italy. *Photo by author.*

periodicals and diurnal papers, it was abandoned in the 1970s and removed and put to rest in the mid-1980s. In the late 1990s, Marco Orlandi an art restorer and citizen of Casalmaggiore—petitioned the town council to have the edicola restored and replaced where it once stood.[77] In July of 2003, the edicola returned to its original location, and its purpose now is to showcase the work of young regional artists. It is what one local reporter referred to as "the world's smallest modern art museum."[78]

This particular cultural icon is among the most notable of its kind because of its unique style.[79] It is a "Liberty" design (taking its name from the art nouveau style inaugurated by the London fashion house of Arthur Lasenby Liberty, popular throughout Europe at the end of the nineteenth century). As Orlandi remarked in a recent interview, the architecture of the Casalmaggiore edicola is especially fitting because although designed with certain distinctive Liberty features

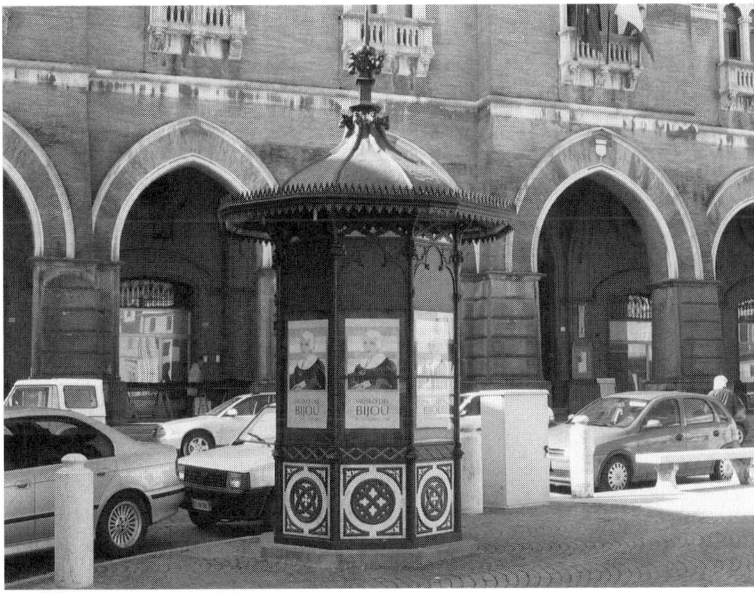

2 Restored Liberty Edicola. *Photo by author.*

such as the minaret-like arches and the bulbous dome, these are done in style with the design of Casalmaggiore's town hall in front of which it sits. Thus, though it was a new structure to the area in 1899 when it was first installed, the present-day edicola in Casalmaggiore repeats the stylistic themes of the town hall while retaining its characteristic art nouveau qualities. Notably, Orlandi explains further, his restoration project was done with this exact purpose in mind: to respect the dialogic contours of the "*arredo urbano*" (urban furniture).[80] Thus with the return of the Liberty edicola of Casalmaggiore, we have "the re-installation of an object whose value is entirely aesthetic so that you have an instance of art occupying a public space."[81] The symmetry between town hall and the restored edicola thus creates a connection between aesthetic value and political value which, according to Orlandi, "recalls how this particular object closely followed for an entire century the most significant events of our city and, from its privileged perch, witnessed the most intense corals of thought, ideological conflict, and the hardships of our citizens."[82]

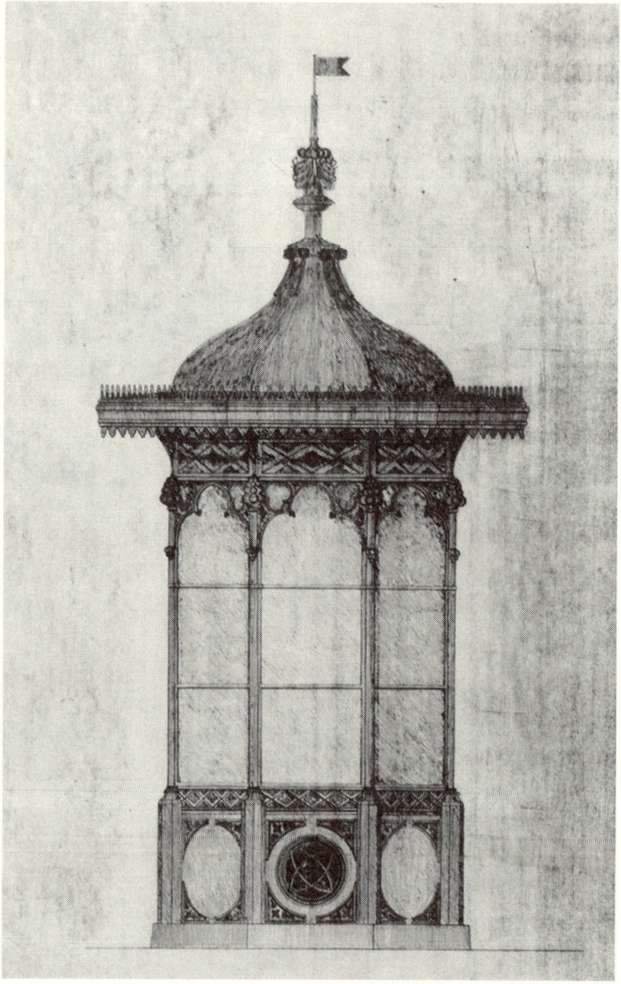

3 Architectural drawing of the Liberty Edicola (1899). Biblioteca Civica A. E. Mortara di Casalmaggiore (with permission). *Photo reproduction by Luigi Briselli.*

Prior to its status as a renovated art object, the edicola had a very specific function: it was the storehouse and mediator of information for the entire town. It was at the edicola that people converged to purchase their daily news, and it was to the windows of the edicola, displaying the news of the day, that people came to read. Those who couldn't read would be captured by the conversations, comments, and remarks circulating around the kiosk. Theirs was an entirely responsive readerly posture that relied on the aural tones emitted by others who read out loud. With the edicola, reading becomes a public event; it creates a space for reading in public where, as one local writer notes, "the secular morning prayer was uttered amongst the passersby who read the daily papers hanging on its windows, allowing the individual reader to become a citizen of the great piazza of the world."[83]

"The act of walking," explains de Certeau, "is to the urban system what the speech act is to language or to statements uttered."[84] With this, de Certeau suggests that the textuality of the urban experience—the zig-zag of walking, the pitter-patter of footsteps, and the composition of paths (*tourner un parcours*)—creates an ethopoesis of space that differs from the idea of a location that one owns or can even call one's own. As a vector of images, sounds, and space, the edicola stands as a kind of political icon that composes trajectories of movement. It is at once a point of convergence and dislocation, it guides the eyes of the reader and occasions the sound of moving lips, read words, and moving bodies. As a source of daily news, Orlandi notes, the edicola "was the physical locus of diurnal information par excellence for at least three generations."[85] And to this we might add that it stood witness to the public events that defined the cultural life of a polity from the proclamation of the Italian Republic in 1946 to the various Po floods that invaded the banks of Casalmaggiore. The edicola is an object of capture and testimony to the noise of utterance.

When Roger Chartier affirms that "reading is not uniquely an abstract operation of the intellect: it brings the body into play,"[86] we are reminded of how the edicola must have contributed to this play of bodies in the reading life of the town of Casalmaggiore. As a newsstand it is a source of information, but to leave it at that would be to

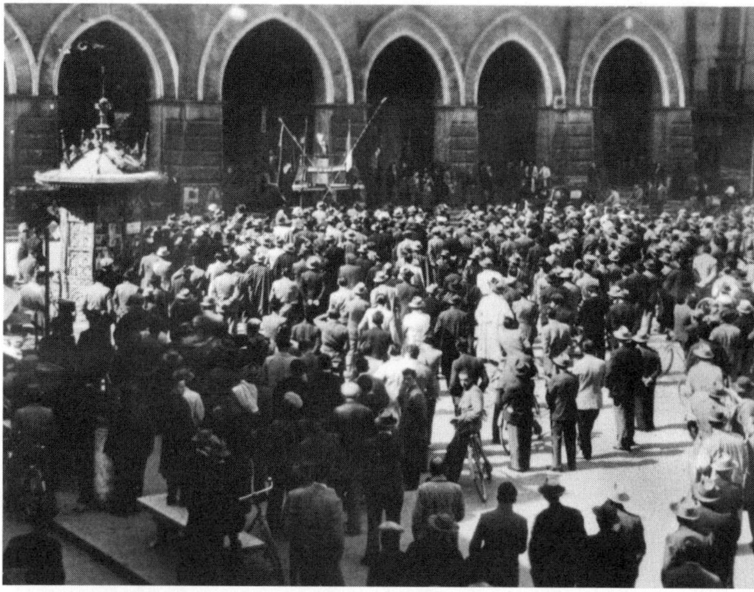

4 Piazza Garibaldi, Casalmaggiore: Proclamation of the Italian Republic (1946) with Liberty Edicola in foreground. Biblioteca Civica A. E. Mortara di Casalmaggiore (with permission). *Photo reproduction by Luigi Briselli.*

overlook the ethopoetic modalities of perceptual attention that this structure occasions: it is a source of conversation, a source of bodily convergence, a source for polemics—in short, an aesthetico-political node of the political life of sensation. With the edicola and the piazza on which it stands, we find an object that at once collects and disseminates the stories of a culture whose regimes of perception are as diverse and clamorous as the individuals constituted by them.

In the division between text and reader, between speaker and listener, we find the materiality of the reading and talking experience that has physical objects like the book, the piazza, and the edicola as its source. This is not to say that without such objects, utterances would be silent, nor is it to say that these are the only objects that occasion noise. It is to say, however, that by extending our conceptions of what counts as sources for political interlocution beyond the grammatical and hermeneutic limits of the semantic statement and the deliberative limits of philosophical argument, we discover modalities of political expression that don't simply rely on the need to communicate sense but also generate noise, like the baking of pre-Directive chocolate. The edicola—its shape, position, and status as newsstand—creates an *"espace lisible"* of what de Certeau refers to as the art of nonsense; "the art of beginning or re-beginning to speak by saying."[87]

To practice this art involves something much more complex than what the epistemic claim has to offer, it beckons a reconsideration of the phonetic aspects of the utterance. The art of nonsense thus finds punctual expression in the noise of the utterance by introducing disjuncture in the supposed unity between harmony and sense. Like Kandinsky's line, or de Certeau's walker, this speech genre traces vectors of movement that interrupt diurnal rhythms. With this aural dimension of speech in mind, the familiar manners of deliberation—tact, politesse, consensus, and so on—cannot account for the art of democratic noise. A theoretical enterprise grounded in the stability of the written word, therefore, always risks circumscribing its analytic acumen to the stenographic representation of democratic culture. This inevitably results in the setting aside of a series of other sounds, noises, and moving traces that, because nongraphic, cannot be counted within the narratocratic armory of political discourse.

Political reflection must leave open the possibility that there is another side to sense—a democratic non-sense—that constitutes a moment of capture in the political life of sensation. To register such aural temporalities, we can turn our attention to forms of observational evidence that retain the sonorous traces of the noise of the utterance: to architectural structures like piazzas, edicolas, and other monuments that help recall the noises people make when saying before stating, when enunciating before making sense. This Babelian moment of saying before stating is a democratic moment par excellence: it is the moment when voice encounters sense, when the correspondences of perception are yet to be secured, offering occasions of part-taking by those whose utterances are not yet speech.

CHAPTER THREE

Machiavelli's Theory of Sensation and Florence's *Vita Festiva*

In an essay from which I draw extensively in these pages, the medieval art critic and theorist Michael Camille footnotes his findings stating that his are the results of "ongoing conversations presented here not as conclusions but as directions for future research."[1] His tragic and untimely death (April 29, 2002 at age forty-four) made it so that his own work could not continue the brilliant trajectory he had set out. Though I never met Michael Camille, in my work I have benefited greatly from his insights and hope the following might add to the many ongoing conversations that his writings have sparked.

Introduction to the *Vita Festiva*

> We must understand that vision is not completed in the eyes. . . . There must be something sentient besides the eyes, in which vision is completed and of which the eyes are the instruments that give it the visible species. ROGER BACON

The arrival of the newspaper edicola in Casalmaggiore's central piazza in the late nineteenth century is a relatively recent event in the political life of sensation. However, as a node of cultural intensities, the edicola's popular history is not as recent. One finds its traces in the early-modern "edicole sacre,"[2] which were kiosks that housed and protected cult artifacts in public spaces. From a sacred image to the possible relic, these little temples offered occasion for the public display of religious faith that accompanied an early-modern commitment to the cultural life of the *vita festiva* (festival life). Specifically, the period between the latter half of the quattrocento and the beginning of the cinquecento "witnessed a dazzling array of spectacular ceremonies which reflected the growing stature of Florence, whose position as the center of a regional state was increasingly recognized locally and throughout the rest of Italy, as well as internationally."[3]

Continuing where my analysis of the nineteenth-century edicola left off, in this chapter I argue that the proliferation of festival culture that took place between the fifteenth and sixteenth centuries influenced Florentine political thought and the theory of sensation that Niccolò Machiavelli develops in his political writings. I begin with a discussion of festival historiography and the historiography of Machiavelli's political thought. I then shift emphasis and look to the political life of sensation that formed the backdrop of the aesthetic and scientific pursuits of the period, and examine how these might have influenced Machiavelli's theory of sensation. I contend that, in order to appreciate the role of festivals in the public life of a political culture, we must distance ourselves from—though not entirely abandon—the conceptual approach to discourse analysis.[4] With this in mind I turn my discussion to Machiavelli's letter to Francesco Vettori (written December 10, 1513) in order to expand on the role of sensation in *The Prince* and, most notably, in chapter 18 ("How Princes Should Keep Faith"). In these pages we see Machiavelli disrupting certain organoleptic assurances by collapsing the distinction between viewing and touching. This collapse, I argue, is crucial to Machiavelli's political thinking both in terms of his commitment to the political life of sensation and to an early-modern rearticulation of the political.

Niccolò's Privilege

To suggest that Machiavelli holds a privileged post in the canon of political thought amounts to stating the obvious. Whether his ideas are viewed within the context of an economy of violence (Wolin), as one of the "waves of modernity" (Strauss), or as purveyor and protector of an ancient Roman republican tradition (Skinner, Pocock, Arendt), Machiavelli's stature in modern political thought is undisputed; so undisputed, in fact, that despite his nefarious reputation (both secular and religious), he remains protected by church walls along with a pantheon of other Florentine figures buried in the Church of Santa Croce in Florence.

As John McCormick has outlined the various tenets of some of the most important achievements of Machiavelli historiography in recent decades, I will refrain from doing the same. But whereas McCormick's essay focuses on the Cambridge school's conceptual analysis of Machiavelli's republicanism and retorts that what they have overlooked is the extra-institutional "active, 'ferocious' defense of popular liberty that is pursued through extra-electoral devices and practices in Machiavelli's 'tribunate' reconstruction of ancient Rome,"[5] I want to proceed with an examination of some of the perceptual assumptions of the Cambridge school's approach.

In the previous chapter I addressed some of these assumptions and, with apologies to the reader, I will rehearse some of these here as they are relevant to the discussion that follows. Cambridge school historiography, I argued, holds a narratocratic commitment to the strict correspondences between sight and reading, touch and writing. In his methodological writings, Quentin Skinner is forthcoming about this, arguing that the task of the historian is to wrestle with words, their uses, and their meanings.[6] If history has an object world, that world is comprised of letters that combine to compose meaningful utterances in the form of speech acts. Thinking, and political and moral theory as special cases of the activity we call thinking, is an enterprise that requires a readerly attention to language. This is what Skinner means when he says that the types of utterances he is interested in can never be viewed simply as strings of propositions but instead as "moves in an argument."[7] Thus, in order to understand the meaning of an utterance qua argument, we must assume that "any act of communication will always constitute the taking up of some determinate position in relation to some pre-existing conversation or argument."[8] The history of political thought is a history of *disputatio* which determines the ideological position of an author that can then be mapped onto a context of other speech utterances.

Working within this same interpretive framework, Maurizio Viroli defends Machiavelli's republican ambitions. Viroli begins with the interpretive dilemma of trying to recover what Machiavelli did with the concept of politics in the hope of adjusting our own understandings of what counts as political phenomena. The point, he continues, is that in our day and age we all rely either implicitly or explicitly on "a Machiavellian understanding of politics as games of power, convenience and self-interest which are to be discussed in the language of empirical science."[9] If we discover that Machiavelli had something else in mind when he was talking about politics, then maybe "we might be tempted to reconsider our mental habits concerning politics."[10] Thus the practice of doing history is employed not only in the service of conceptual clarification but also as a way of staging a clash of convictions between accurate and inaccurate accounts of politics. To achieve such a staging, Viroli advises a strategy: "start by describing the conventional ways of speaking about politics in the literature of his [i.e., Machiavelli's] time."[11]

Here we have an explicit collapsing of the distinction between reading, writing, and speaking that is invoked in order to clarify the concepts of a particular author. Written words are a kind of speaking, they involve a posture of address and a readerly attention that, when accurately understood, allows us to determine the normative elements of a theorist's ideas. But in the case of Viroli's investigation, something much more dramatic occurs. Through a careful and striking analysis of the political lexicon available to a Florentine public, he shows how Machiavelli's *The Prince* could not be viewed as a political tract by the author himself because the kind of language Machiavelli uses in *The Prince* does not correspond to the conventional language of politics at the time. Most of the vocabulary of politics, Viroli explains, is borrowed from Aristotle. But here we have a thoroughly romanized Aristotle thanks to Leonardo Bruni's translation of the philosopher's texts. It was Bruni's translations that made the shift from the Greek language of *politia* to the Latin *civitas* possible and through this shift, "the image of the city is expressed in a vocabulary that becomes predominant in Renaissance humanist political literature. The *civitas* is much more than the source of protection and the supplier of material needs, it is the humane community where the citizens have in common laws, magistracies, and religious and public ceremonies. In a true city," Viroli concludes, "the relationships between citizens are relationships of friendship and solidarity."[12]

This shift in vocabulary makes it so that politics and *civitas* become indistinct. More importantly, the literary reconfiguration of public life from *politia* to *civitas* also implies a shift in moral habits; now individuals no longer consider themselves as singular entities but view themselves as citizens of a city, and thus as responsible for the well-ordering of that space. Politics, Viroli concludes, "circulated within the confines of the city; outside the city or against civil life politics had no place."[13] To be sure, it is not simply the practice of politics that circulates within the confines of the city, it is also and especially the vocabulary of *politia* as *civitas* that circulates within these walls. That is, the words themselves are bearers of a *vivere civile* that require the "habits of civic virtue"[14] in order for liberty to be maintained.

It may seem pedantic to exploit the image of language that Viroli relies on; but it isn't because it's precisely through the insistence on the impact of vocabulary, of the fact that language impacts our sensory perceptions, that we can endorse its capacity to create a new morphology of moral habits. And it is the organoleptic dimensions of *iter*-impact that make it possible for Viroli's analysis of Machiavelli's republicanism to make any sense at all. The vocabulary of *civitas*, like the ball in a squash court, bounces back and forth only within the walls of the city. Whatever happens outside the city, Viroli wants to insist, cannot be allegorized in terms of either *politia* or *civitas*. Thus it is that Machiavelli "never uses the word *politico* or its equivalent in *The Prince*."[15] And the reason for this is that in *The Prince* "he simply was not writing about politics as he understood the term."[16] In avoiding the term *"politico"* in *The Prince* and referring to the treatise as a work in the *arte dello stato* (as he does in his letter to Vettori, written December 10, 1513), Machiavelli is actually enacting his republican commitments by safeguarding the terms of *politico* discourse. The *arte dello stato*, Viroli concludes, "is not the same as the art of the city because the *stato* is not the equivalent of the *civitas* or the *vivere politico*."[17] If *The Prince* is not a treatise on "politics" as Machiavelli would have understood the term, then the exiled secretary's republican commitments are well insured and we, too, can be secure in the thought that "Machiavelli's deepest love was for those who possessed the art of instituting a political life."[18]

I am less concerned with the republican image of Machiavelli that Viroli projects than I am with the move he makes in limiting the scope of the *vivere politico* in order to defend Machiavelli's conception of *libertas*. For, in doing so, he not only limits what is available to political reflection—namely vocabulary—but he also partitions what is available to political experience (i.e., the boundaries of city walls). In short, it's not simply the case that political action takes place in the city, it is also the case that what we recognize as political will be so if and only if it corresponds to a way of reading typographical inscriptions determined by a narratocratic regime of perception. If an act is not describable within the terms of the specific morphology of the vivere civile thusly derived, like the *arte dello stato*, then it is not political and is not sympathetic with political reflection.

Florence's *Vita Festiva*

The growing culture of republican virtues in Renaissance Italy, John Pocock explains, begins with a literary reconfiguration of a historical archetype. The equivocal figure in this regard is Brutus and his stature as political hero or villain. Here is Pocock: "Dante had seen Brutus as a traitor against his superior, and since that superior prefigured the emperor, who reigned over the hierarchies of men as did God over the hierarchies of nature, had placed him and Cassius beside Judas who had betrayed God himself. But the subsequent revolution in historical imagery presented Brutus as the type of republican citizen and tyrannicide, and condemned Caesar as tyrant and subverter of the republic."[19] The repositioning of Brutus from damned soul to popular hero is, to be sure, a textual one; but it is also one that speaks volumes not only about Florentine attitudes regarding republicanism but, more importantly, to their obsession with image creation.

Indeed, the pontifical stature of the vocabulary of *libertas* in much republican historiography is equivocal at best within the context of a world of appearances. It may be true that the inscription "*Libertas*" still survives hanging over Palazzo Vecchio in Florence, but as Alison Brown points out, the persistence of this icon is no indication of the iconic stature of the concept itself. Rather, the *dimostrazione* (appearance) of the word "liberty" may be just that, "a role-playing function in representing—or mis-representing—the image of 'liberty' in Florence."[20] The fact is that a commitment to liberty as a political ideal is secure if—and only if—we limit our considerations to the ideational properties of the concept of liberty.

As much as the years between the quattrocento and cinquecento may have been an intense period of political thought, they were also marked by an explosion of imagery and an equally explosive commitment to the public circulation of images. And this commitment to sensorial impact came with an awareness of the relationship between artifice and dissemblance. Pier Filippo Pandolfini, Lorenzo de' Medici's ambassador to Rome, perhaps stated the matter best when, in accounting for the Pope's sincerity, had this to say in a letter dated February 4, 1487: "in these times things are judged more so on the basis of their effects rather than on the meaning of words."[21] Melissa Bullard treats such pronouncements as a "crisis" in image making and as expressing an anxiety about the dissimulating power of the image, what she refers to as "the real drama of people's desperate attempts to cover the yawning gap between language and reality" that lay behind "the façade of theatricality."[22] But this seems like a premature conclusion, especially given the fact that there was such an active and popular participation in image making. Thus, though people were aware of the tensions between image and reality, and may have sought to discriminate between an individual's appearance and their deeds, they were nonetheless committed to creating "*effetti*."

More to the point, it seems that just as Florentines were aware of the relationship between the image and its effects, they were equally aware of the ways in which the correspondences between image and effect were far from secure; one might even go so far as to suggest that they were indistinct. One case in particular marks this point well: the Palm Sunday procession of 1496. It was conceived by Savonarola, and it was, like every other similar festive event, "planned by both friar and government to ensure its emotional success."[23] The procession is a carefully scripted, mapped, and controlled event and though paradisiacal enthusiasm is an emotion that might arise out of it, we cannot isolate enthusiasm as the sole emotion and certainly not its principal objective.

By all accounts, the Palm Sunday procession was a success to the extent that the participants sang great lauds, were moved to dance, and as Richard Trexler describes it, to "tearfully loving the other in a craze of fraternity."[24] At this point, amid the song, dance, and ringing of church bells, the brethren started chanting "*Viva Cristo!*" A "Hurray for Christ!" might at first seem entirely innocent given the rapture that gripped the brethren. But the "*Viva Cristo!*" was exclaimed on Palm Sunday, the day in the Church calendar when Christ's *trionfo* (triumph), his entering into Jerusalem, is at once celebrated and remembered as the event that precedes his betrayal. The brethren's "*Viva Cristo!*" was thus also an interruptive moment in the celebration that must have created a panic among the official organizers. Were the brethren chanting in enthusiastic support of the Christ figure or were they participating in an impromptu moment of "*sacra rappresentazione*,"[25] ironically siding with those who lauded Jesus with palms on one day only to crown him with thorns the next?

Moreover, the "*viva*," like the "*Libertas*" on Palazzo Vecchio, when spoken rather than read, marks an excess of enthusiasm. It is a battle cry of allegiance at the cost of all else, a hyperbole of conviction.[26] The equivocal stature of the noise of the "*viva!*" points to what Trexler refers to as the "fundamentally contradictory attitude"[27] of festive forms more generally, especially in times of political instability. The exuberance of the organized procession at once relaxes tensions by creating an outlet for public enthusiasm, but also creates further tensions—equivocations of attachment, if you will—when noises like the *"viva!"* resound.

The 1496 Palm Sunday procession is a relatively late example of Florence's *vita festiva*. Indeed, it comes after a period of stasis in the public life of Florence imposed by the Medici family after the Pazzi Conspiracy (1478).[28] Prior to that stasis, however, no figure stands out as more encouraging and more controversial in the proliferation of popular festive forms than Lorenzo de' Medici. As many have remarked, Lorenzo's title of magnificence (and the culture of magnificence more generally associated with him) was the result of his own manufacture; Lorenzo was a master craftsmen when it came to producing the right effects for his own image.[29] Successfully surviving the Pazzi Conspiracy (unlike his unfortunate brother, Giuliano), Lorenzo designed a medal to be struck in Florence to commemorate the event, with his face on one side under the inscription *"salus publica"* (health of the people) and that of his brother on the other with the inscription *"luctus publicus"* (grief of the people). That there could be a connection to the mythical Romulus and Remus, with Lorenzo as the "brother who survived to carry on the destiny of his people" was certainly not lost on his contemporaries, nor on succeeding generations.[30]

Lorenzo's capacity for such forms of arresting image making were also expressed through his involvement in Florence's popular festive life.[31] But here, disagreement persists regarding the intent of these events. On the one hand, scholars like Paola Ventrone argue that "the production of spectacles was a communal event, deeply rooted in social practice, which constantly fluctuated between the private behavior of the promoting groups—such as confraternities, guild corporations, and neighborhood congregations—and the public, civic displays of these same groups, thus revealing the status of these groups to be at once 'public' and 'private'."[32] On the other, Nicole Carew-Reid insists on the negative reading, claiming that "the festivities in Florence of the Fifteenth Century may be interpreted as a double-edged societal affirmation of a celebration of the established powers. They were greater and greater tributes to the personalities of the directors who would manipulate their elements in order to acquire personal prestige."[33]

Carew-Reid's study is especially persuasive. Her readings of Lorenzo's text of the sacra rappresentazione in 1491, which took place during that year's carnival festivities, show the extent to which Lorenzo insists on self-aggrandizing themes of glory, power, and obedience by the people. And some might say that these elements are also present in Lorenzo's carnival writings, the oft-cited *Canti Carnascialeschi*, where behind the carpe diem themes in songs like the "Canzone di Bacco" one might find a heavy-handed Lorenzo wanting to impose his own image of greatness through writing and song.[34] However, as Ventrone retorts, the emphasis on the sacra rappresentazione of 1491 is ambiguous and misleading since this is only one of two festivities in which Lorenzo participated directly; thus suggesting that rather than showing Lorenzo's attempt at what Carew-Reid refers to as "seduction through spectacle," it reveals "the ambiguities and weaknesses of Lorenzo's position as ruler."[35]

More than the ambiguities and weaknesses of Lorenzo's position, it reveals the ambiguities and equivocations of festival life itself.[36] The inversion of the figure of Brutus from traitor to hero in Leonardo Bruni's (1361–1444) writings cited by Pocock is accompanied by the equivocal status of Lorenzo's own image as either *salus publica* or tyrant and, indeed, by the equivocality of the "effetti" of the vocabulary of "*libertas*" and the noise of the "*viva!*" These equivocations—what Bakhtin characterizes as the ambivalences of highs and lows characteristic of popular festive forms—do not so much speak to an accurate representation of the culture of the vita festiva as to the difficulty with which a conceptual approach to history can assess the culture of appearance that pervades the political life of sensation between the end of the quattrocento and the beginning of the cinquecento.

Intromission and Machiavelli's Theory of Sensation

The *Canti Woodcut* (see figure 5) represents a carnival scene.[37] The five young men dressed in festive garb, two of whom are holding a doughnut-like pastry traditionally eaten at carnival, stand beneath a

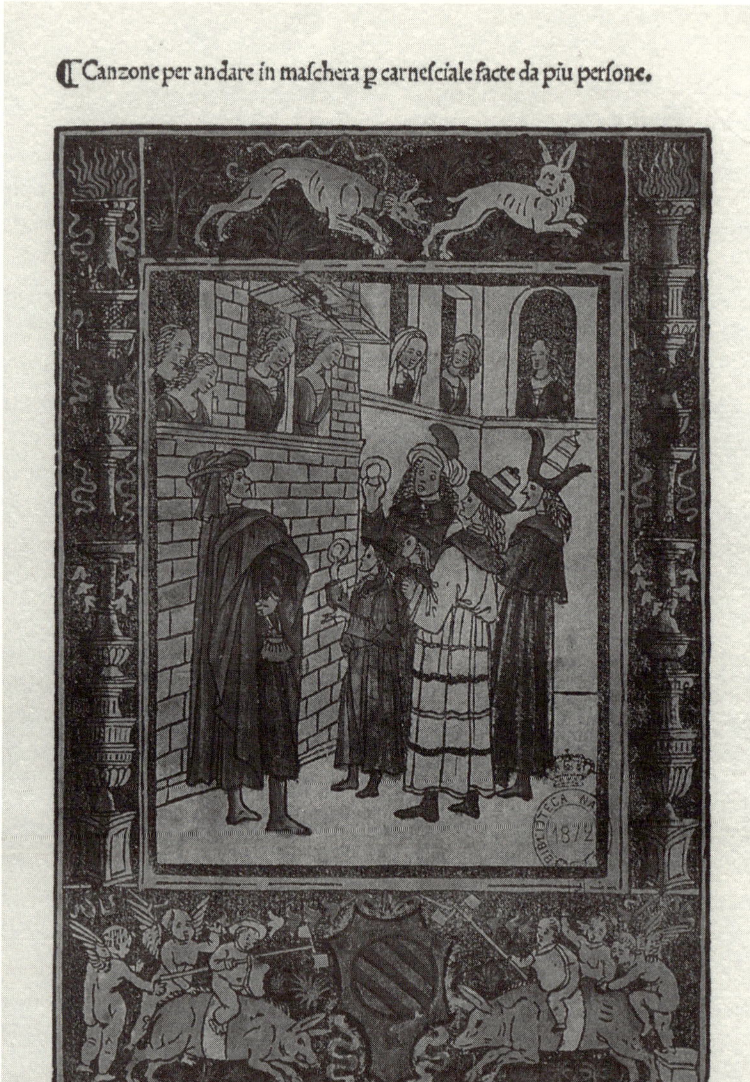
Canzone per andare in maſchera p carneſciale facte da piu perſone.

5 Sixteenth-century woodcut of Florentine carnival scene in *Trionfi e canti carnascialeschi toscani del Rinascimento,* edited by Riccardo Bruscagli.

row of windows singing to the women perched on the window sills. The women look down toward the men and seem pleased by the display of courtship. Framing the woodcut are typical images of marginalia: at the top of the page a wolflike hound chases a rabbit with some concupiscence; on the sides there are ornate columns bearing the weight of the scene; and on the bottom, a representation of the simultaneity of the sacred and profane characteristic of carnival, with cherubim riding what seem like wild boar, enacting one of the more popular games of the vita festiva, the joust. If, as Michael Camille states, "one of the most powerful statements that the monstrosities of marginal art make is that they violate the taboo that separates the human from the animal,"[38] then in the case of the *Canti Woodcut* there is a notable extension of this taboo: animal and divine are intermingled, playing together in a clumsy but comical fashion.

Curious as these images may have been, the most curious figure is the one standing to the side. Neither participating in singing, nor expressing pleasure in the songs themselves, he stares sternly at the men. His fashion differs from theirs: he is cloaked, wears a turban, and carries a purse. It's almost as if he governs the scene with both his eyes as well as his purse strings. And indeed he might. The figure has been linked to Lorenzo and to the controversial role he might have played in the public life of Florence's vita festiva. That debate seems less relevant, though, than the visual play of capture in this carnival scene. It's almost as if Lorenzo's visual posture is a representation not only of wealth and power but of a kind of attitude toward language: to wit, the princely figure standing at the edge governs the correct use of language. Lorenzo wants to make sure that the songs are being sung well precisely because he is their author. Here the sovereigntist image of princely power and control comes from a commitment to seeing words used correctly; to making sure, from an appropriate though not invisible distance, that the singers' cant is in the right tone. Riccardo Bruscagli's introduction to this edition of *Canzone per andare in maschera* makes the point succinctly: "Savonarola's 'tyrant', suggestively distinguishable also by the richness of his wardrobe, is not merely the *auctor* who follows with paternal affection the *iter* of his creatures: he is also the lord who controls the developments of a pre-ordained festival, who rules both internally and in the first person, the use of 'popular' linguistic and sociological categories, of which he is their first and paradoxical creator."[39] From this, one might go so far as to suggest that the desire to direct language, its usage, and its reception—the image of language as disputatio—is one of the most princely of all images of language.[40]

Fundamental to the operation of the "iter," as Bruscagli describes it, is the organoleptic claim that words have impacts, that they are part of the percept world, and that their influence extends well beyond the written script. Indeed, this woodcut invokes a carnival context of sensation that is not simply about emotions or passions. Emotions and passions, though occupying an important role in our experiential life, exist within a regime of perception where the partitions of the sensible are already well established. But, what the discourse on the passions does not do is allow us to question the value of these partitions (because they are the given that legislate the possibility of sense): to imagine these divisions as constitutive of political reflection (the prereflective that enables reflection) means that we tacitly acknowledge a consensus regarding perceptual experience and organization.

From the perspective of a theory of sensation—one that, as Brian Massumi has shown, implies a "cofunctioning" of vision with other senses[41]—these narratocratic assumptions become problematic. Here we can no longer rely on a readerly repose of thought because it is not the construction of the sentence as it is written and as it is presumed spoken that matters. This, of course, does not imply a rejection of narrative tout court. It simply asserts that there are different levels at which perception operates and that the linearity of narrative emplotment is only one—among many—regimes of perception.

How, then, might the perceptual shift from sense making to sensation assist us in our inquiry into the role of Florence's vita festiva in Machiavelli's political thought? At a very basic level, and as the abundance of research into the public life of Renaissance Florence shows, this was a period oddly committed to the life of sensation, to the proliferation of intensities impacting the body. This was also a time when developments in artistic competencies corresponded to profound alterations in the life of perception. Most famously, Brunelleschi's discovery of the vanishing point in perspective, arrived at through a series of experiments that involved a mirror, a pinhole, and Florence's baptistery (c. 1425),[42] is a case in point. This innovation not only resulted in a revolutionary change in the world of painting—what some modern commentators refer to as the discovery of the distinction between the visual world and the visual field—but it also resulted in a radical shift in regimes of perception.[43] Now, with the capacity to paint a scene with geometric proportions (by starting from a central point on the canvas that represents the point at which the lines of visuality converge), we arrive at the realization that the source of unity in perception is not the outside world but our own vision of it; a realization made explicit by Brunelleschi's conclusion that "the visual axis, when directed straight ahead, determines the horizon—and therefore the single, unifying vanishing point."[44] But in order for this to work, we must imagine a reciprocal relation between our postures of visual attention and our perception of the world. When our posture shifts, so does the axis of the vanishing point, and thus also what is available to attention. Moreover, we must assume that though the construction of proportion in a painting is possible, this visual field is entirely artificial since linear perspective relies on the difference between the visual world and the visual field. Finally, what Brunelleschi's discovery also assumes is a theory of sensation—*intromission*—that had been in play for several centuries.[45]

St. Augustine had championed *extromission*—or, the idea that the object world was produced by the act of viewing.[46] Unlike Brunelleschi's viewing—which relies on artifice as the basis of proportion—Augustine's viewing emphasized the power of the image itself over the will of the individual (e.g., the eyes of cultish statues that captured the spectator). On this view, a visual fire emanates from our eyes and combines with the aura of the object. Hence the Neoplatonic admonitions against the world of images and the reliable cohesion of the world of the senses with cupidity in Augustine. For him, the senses were dangerous because they reached out to the world of images, as it were, embracing the potential for sin. However, as Michael Camille shows through an analysis of a medieval diagram representing cognition, a shift occurs in medieval practices of seeing from extromission to intromission. Rather than emphasizing how the object is generated by the spectator's view, intromission "placed the world of nature and the world of art on the same footing, as objects of sense, bringing the outside world in."[47] Here the flow of intensity is reversed, emphasizing the impact of objects on the body.

Now we enter the world of impressions (Camille cites Aquinas's use of Aristotle's metaphor of the wax seal to describe sensation); moreover, we enter a dynamic world where the intervening spaces between individual bodies and objects matter; finally, we enter into a world where objects impact our bodies and where the intensity of such impacts makes it difficult to distinguish between the affected senses. Indeed, "intromission placed the world of nature in a new relation to the viewer as objects of sense that could be known."[48] At once, it took for granted the fact that the image created in the mind—what was referred to as the *sensus communis vel sensatio*—is the result of "a compound image of the external sensed object, often combining more than one sense."[49]

We can begin to grasp the importance of this theory of sensation when we consider how, knowing that sensatio is a compound, Brunelleschi had to revert to the pinhole experiment to "discover" the vanishing point. That is, it is on the basis of a theory of sensation rooted in intromission that Brunelleschi was able to create a visual field of reflection (literally using a mirror). Balanced proportion, so important to Renaissance theories of perception and indeed to Western aesthetics writ large, is ultimately the result of an experiment that partitions sensation by isolating the visual field. Yet what Brunelleschi's experiment does not isolate, because it relies on it, is the force of intromission. The pinhole circumscribes the experiential field, but not the intensity of the image impacting the mirror.

Niccolò Machiavelli lived and wrote in a time when intromission structured people's perceptual competencies, and the secretary's commitment to this is nowhere more evident than in his account of what Miguel Vatter has recently called Machiavelli's "theory of the *riscontro*."[50] Riscontro (encounter, clash, or impact), Vatter explains, sources Machiavelli's critique of prudential logic. More to the point, the theory of the *riscontro* shows that human "nature" is a function of habits of action acquired thanks to the favor bestowed by circumstances on a given way of proceeding, i.e., thanks to the adaptation of these ways to the times. Human "nature" in Machiavelli is a function of custom, it is always "second nature." If human "nature" is not something given, but a result of a certain adaptation between actions and circumstances, it is possible to conceive of a mode of action that is not "natural" or "customary," a mode of action that Machiavelli calls "extra-ordinary virtù" (*istraordinaria virtù*) precisely because it goes counter to customary activity. This kind of action goes against customary activity in the sense that it coincides (*riscontro*) with the active changing of the times, whereas customary activity is constituted by the very prohibition of such a coincidence, by remaining always in a position of passivity with respect to the possibility of such changes of time.[51]

Vatter's concern is to explain how Machiavelli deals with the central problem of *fortuna*; namely, that the same action might be successful in one instant and an utter failure the next. Machiavelli's exaltation of *istraordinaria virtù*, he concludes, rests on the fact that Fortuna is an intensity that interrupts a "given way of proceeding," that impacts customary activity, and that such a coincidence of forces necessitates a mode of acting that cannot rely on a preordained regime of perception.

In Vatter's explanation of Machiavelli's theory of the riscontro, then, we find all the elements of an intromission-based theory of sensation that cannot be divorced from the life of the vita festiva. Recall the impact generated by the noise of the "*Viva Cristo!*" or, indeed, the belief that images are sources of effetti (e.g., the "*Libertas*" hanging in Palazzo Vecchio but also the contentious role of Lorenzo as both "tyrant" and salus publica). These examples point to a world of invisible forces that impact (riscontro) our bodies generating sensations. The quality of the man with "extra-ordinary virtù" is a quality based on the ability to engage the riscontro of sensation that occurs in the diurnal life of the vita festiva—the public life where the intermingling of highs and lows creates zones of indistinction that circumscribe the guarantees of prudence, habit, or custom as reliable guideposts for action. But more to the point, Machiavelli's "extraordinary virtù" is the virtù of not expecting our perceptive competencies to always function in the same manner; this is the virtù of realizing that the partitions of the sensible and the corresponding organization of the body is temporary, that political reflection does indeed require a regime of perception, but that the condition of riscontro makes it so that what counts as an organized way of seeing is provisionally determined by this encounter.

For his treatment of Machiavelli's theory of the riscontro, Vatter turns to the text known as the *Ghiribizzi al Soderino*, written in Perugia in September 1506 and addressed to a nephew of Piero Soderini, the Gonfaloniere (flagbearer), of the Florentine republic. However, I would argue that this theory of sensation forms the basis for Machiavelli's reflections on the *vivere civile*, and it reappears in his later writings as well. Consider the letter to Francesco Vettori, written December 10, 1513:[52] riscontro here is subtle but explicit if we part company with the conventional historiographical partition between the social and political life of Florence.

Recent studies have situated this letter within a larger framework of epistolary writing that carries both Petrarchan and Boccaccian elements.[53] In this regard, Stella Larosa notes that "from this perspective, the two types of 'readings' completed by Machiavelli, the daily one and the nocturnal one, must be analyzed alongside one another, despite the differences that distinguish them."[54] The traditional reading, and the one that Larosa ultimately sustains despite suggesting a parallelism, is that the contrast between the diurnal events comprising Machiavelli's time in exile and the nocturnal encounters with ancient men represents a break between the banality and depression of his social existence and the vitality of a fantastical world of political and intellectual engagement. Here is Machiavelli's famous description:

> On the coming of evening, I return to my house and enter my study; and at the door I take off the day's clothing, covered with mud and dust, and put on garments regal and courtly; and reclothed appropriately, I enter the ancient courts of ancient men, where, received by them with affection, I feed on the food which only is mine and which I

> was born for, where I am not ashamed to speak with them and to ask them the reason for their actions; and they in their kindness answer me; and for four hours of time I do not feel boredom, I forget every trouble, I do not dread poverty, I am not frightened by death; entirely I give myself over to them.[55]

The notes he takes from these conversations, he goes on to explain, are "fantasies," meticulously transcribed and transformed into "a little work *On Princedoms*." The passage is striking, particularly in contrast with the previous two paragraphs where Machiavelli explains how his day begins with having to cut wood, followed by a period of reading by a stream (Dante or Petrarch or one of the "lesser poets, such as Tibullus, Ovid, and the like"—to wit, authors Savonarola had condemned)[56]; he then visits his local inn where he speaks "with those who pass, ask news of their villages, learn various things, and note the various tastes and different fancies of men." After dinner he returns to the inn and with the host, a butcher, a miller, and two furnace tenders, he "sinks into vulgarity for the whole day, playing at *cricca* and at trich-trach, and then these games bring on a thousand disputes and countless insults with offensive words . . . So," he concludes the paragraph prior to the one cited above, "mixed up with these lice, I keep my brain from growing moldy."[57]

The contrast *is* notable, to say the least; and, as already mentioned, the pleasure with which Machiavelli describes his nocturnal habits is made even more spectacular in contrast to the baseness of the diurnal engagements.[58] But contrast does not necessarily imply negation for there doesn't seem to be anything in the contrast that suggests that the two moments are mutually exclusive or dialectically opposed. To be sure, Machiavelli is far from content with what has happened to him; indeed, he is miserable. But he is not miserable because he has to spend time in the inn. On the contrary, inn-life helps keep his brain "from growing moldy." Everything about this scene, in other words, implies a life of sensation and riscontro. He cuts wood (the riscontro of the axe upon the tree); this results in a dispute (a riscontro over cordage, theft, and so forth); upon leaving the grove, he engages in a literary riscontro by a stream with indexed poets; at the inn, he encounters (riscontro) travelers and, like the notes he takes with ancient men that compose his "little work *On Princedoms*," he takes notes on "the various tastes and different fancies of men." He then dines (a riscontro on the palate), feeding on shared peasant food (only to then enter his home and continue to "feed on that food which only is mine"), and of course he engages in a series of physical and aural riscontri while playing games at the inn.

With all these riscontri in play, it is telling that Larosa's way of describing the difference between the two phases of Machiavelli's day concentrates on the reading rather than the food metaphor. Focusing on the eyes in the event of reading, however, might make us miss the extent to which there is an ambivalent complementarity between the two phases of his day (rather than simply a parallel) that becomes pellucid when we consider the images of consumption, ingestion, and digestion that the food metaphor allows. Now the mouth and the stomach are privileged over the eyes and the mind; or, more accurately, the complementarity of these two moments underlines an indistinction of the eyes with the mouth and stomach.

From the perspective of a culture of eating characteristic of the vita festiva,[59] the riscontri that occur during the day are, for Machiavelli, a moment in the care of the self that prepare him for the nocturnal riscontri.[60] The repetition of the food metaphor suggests the extent to which the distinctions of the quality of the substance consumed (peasant food versus the food of the ancients) are ambivalent and require a cofunctioning of vision with other senses. This point is made even more emphatic if we consider that the food metaphor insists on the ambivalence of the mouth as a source of both speech and mastication. Moreover, silent reading was not as pervasive a textual attitude as it is today. Though we have no way of knowing whether Machiavelli's nocturnal delights were cacophonous or not, we can discern that the ambivalence of the mouth as a source of multiple modes of sensation would not have been lost on him, especially given the rituals of eating during the vita festiva that play on the ambivalence of the mouth as a complex organ designed to consume both the flesh of meat and the body of Christ. (I will have more to say on the ambivalence of the mouth as an organ of political reflection in chapter 5).

In its commitment to representing repeated instances of riscontro throughout the day and night, the letter to Vettori underlines the extent to which the final riscontro with "the ancient courts of ancient men" is one that can occur because of the political life of sensation afforded by the day's more base riscontri. To be sure, Machiavelli emphasizes how he discards his day's clothing "covered in mud and dust." But even this act need not be read as a rejection of the day's events. Rather, like the riscontri in the inn, this is the last stage of his preparation. The sartorial alterations correspond to "the active changing of the times" (Vatter, *Between Form and Event*) which, in the literary structure of the letter is represented by the movement from day to night, from poverty to wealth, from low to high; to wit, central themes of Florence's vita festiva. My point, finally, is that the "entering into the study" can be read as a break from the day only if we assume that the divisions between night and day were crystalline for Machiavelli. Within a regenerative cosmology of the vita festiva, it is not certain that Machiavelli respected such partitions.[61]

That scholars situate *The Prince* within a context of admiration of princes—or, more precisely, "mirror-for-Princes"—should, at this point, not be surprising.[62] However, *The Prince* falls under the category of "mirror-for-Princes" not simply because there is a literary and linguistic context, but because the resplendence of the prince's aura implied in the metaphor of the mirror (that we already saw was crucial to Brunelleschi's studies on linear perspective, vision, and sensation) is one that recalls the political life of sensation of the vita festiva. As the letter to Vettori states, *The Prince* is a text intended to display how a prince should act in order to retain his power. But *The Prince* is also and in every respect an attempt to deal with how it is that the impact (riscontro) of an appearance might be sustained given the fact that the prince is not always visible; the problem of *The Prince*, in other words, is one that speaks to Machiavelli's theory of sensation and to the effetti of invisibility as sources of sensation in a veritable theatrocracy of images. Machiavelli's preoccupation, in short, is with how to sustain the intensive impact of an invisible presence: How can a prince, in his physical absence, continue to appear?

Machiavelli offers a variety of answers to this problem but none have been as controversial as those admonitions found in chapter 18, "How a Prince Should Keep Faith." "A Prince should, therefore, understand how to use well both the man and the beast."[63] The ability a prince has to use both natures, the bestial and the human, is a festival theme now familiar to us and made explicit in the marginalia of the *Canti Woodcut* discussed previously. What has preoccupied thinkers throughout the centuries—and what has made "Machiavellianism" such a negative term—is precisely this commitment to both the human and animal instincts and the suggestion that the skill of the prince rests in the art of "simulating and dissembling."[64]

Machiavelli knows well that "men in general judge rather by the eye than by the hand, for every one can see but few can touch,"[65] and part of what I am suggesting is that one of Machiavelli's concerns throughout his political writings is to insist on the ambivalence between viewing and touching. (I will have more to say about contemporary concerns regarding this ambivalence in the following chapter.) Thus, whatever moral marker one may use to judge Machiavelli's advice to princes, the domain of sensation is the domain within which he (both Machiavelli and the prince) is operating. And though some (e.g., Viroli) may say that this is not a domain of politics because, in *The Prince*, he is not discussing the vivere civile, this seems like an inadequate response given the extent to which the vita festiva and the vivere civile were inextricably linked in Machiavelli's own imaginary. For, though the utterances used to express the difference between "*stato*" and "*vivere civile*" might have different etymological and, indeed, conceptual sources, the reversion to the sensation of riscontro throughout the letter and *The Prince* makes these distinctions problematic at best.

The basis for Machiavelli's account of political life, then, rests on a theory of sensation (intromission) that extends throughout his oeuvre, constituting his central political problematic in *The Prince* and elsewhere: namely, how is it that the intensity of an impression may be sustained in the absence of any physical source? For answers to this, Machiavelli turns to the world of images, ritual, and public life which are, for him and others in the period, part and parcel of the world of politics. Just as we cannot make such a clean division between the passage from day to night in the letter, so are the partitions between the life of the vita festiva and the vivere civile equally indistinct, and their indistinction is afforded by the political life of sensation.

Machiavelli's turn to the sensation of riscontro and the experience of impact in political life is a significant moment in a genealogy of political reflection that compels us to confront the ways in which our ideational life is composed of disjunctive intensities flowing against and through us. But in order to surmise the work of sensation on reflection we must reconsider our received modes of theoretical attention. As significant as the innovations of a narratocratic regime of perception are for a historically inflected approach to the analysis of conceptual artistry, they remain inattentive to their own assumptions about what counts as valuable for political and theoretical reflection. As we saw in the case of Machiavelli's own aesthetic achievements (in both the letter to Vettori and *The Prince*), there is something more at stake there than a sensus communis about the operation of language.[66] There is language at work, of this there is no doubt, but there is also an attentiveness to how organolepsis shares in the ambivalence of the vita festiva so that the stature of the eye as a source of intromission and that of the mouth as an organ of expression are not secure. With such an emphasis on organoleptic indistinction, the vision of language as unified speech flow and the associated image of "theory" as conceptual clarification become problematic at best when engaging Machiavelli's debt to the political life of sensation. Indeed, as we shall see in the subsequent chapters, the status of the mouth and eyes as organs of political reflection continue to raise questions in contemporary debates in political theory, especially with regard to the relationship between citizenship, subjectivity, and the circulation of images in pluralist democracies.

CHAPTER FOUR

The Viewing Subject

Caravaggio, Bacon, and *The Ring*

> The mind is a kind of theatre, where several perceptions successively make their appearance; pass, re-pass, glide away, and mingle in an infinite variety of postures and situations. DAVID HUME

"A blurred shadow. What we have here is the persistence of vision. And as you watch, don't you get an incredible sense of immediacy, as if you're actually a participant in the scene?" This is the conclusion the character Ryuji reaches after viewing the cryptic and disturbing series of images in Koji Suzuki's novel *The Ring* that is the basis for the hugely successful Japanese *Ringu* trilogy as well as its American counterparts, *The Ring* and *The Ring Two*.[1] Ryuji continues: "There are things we see with our eyes, but there are also scenes we conjure up in our minds. And since these don't pass through the retina, there's no blinking involved. But when we actually look with our eyes the images are formed according to the strength of the light that hits the retina. And to keep the retina from drying out, we blink, unconsciously. The black curtain is the instant when the eyes shut."[2]

This explanation comes at a crucial moment in the novel when Ryuji and Asakawa (the main character, an investigative journalist and father whose wife and child have also seen the tape) begin to understand that the film they have been exposed to, and hence the virus that has infected them and that will kill them within a week's time, is not simply a camera recording. Indeed, as Ryuji insists in a thoroughly Humean fashion, what they've viewed and become participant in through this viewing is a mental image imprinted on the filmic patina. The crucial component in this discovery, however, is not the progression of images at all but "the black curtain" made noticeable when the film is slowed down and its successive stream interrupted. The black curtain is the blink, an irrational cut made palpable when the eyes shut.[3] It is this crucial insight that shocks the main characters to the point of nausea. What they are viewing is not so much a succession of images but the process of celluloid impression as it occurs in the mind of the filmmaker. It is a moment of haptic visuality that differs in important ways from mere seeing.

The filmmaker in the novel, it turns out, is a young woman (Sadako Yamamura) who was raped and murdered by the last man in Japan to have been exposed to the smallpox virus; after raping her, he disposes of her by throwing her in a well.[4] The combination of the shock of the rape, the moment of death, the moment of viral infection, and the documented telekinetic powers of Sadako combine in an instance of release (one could even say of birth) so violent and fantastical that the last things that pass through her mind become impressed on the "pestilential videotape."[5] It might seem, then, that the point of the novel and subsequently the first movie (*Ringu* and *The Ring*) is to unveil, witness to, and recount this moment of impression. After all, the narrative appears to be a subgenre of detective fiction. But this conclusion could be true if and only if we were to remain in a regime of visuality governed by an allegorical reading of the plot. Yet, the themes of filmic exposure and viral infection through viewing—and, indeed, the fact that what "cures" the curse is not the discovery of and witnessing to murder but rather the reproduction and dissemination of the film—complicate if not negate entirely the narratocratic approach. Asakawa is explicit about this: "No video camera recorded those images," he explains, "Those images are things that Sadako saw with her eyes and things she imagined in her head, fragments presented one after another with nothing to contextualize them."[6] It's almost as if the narrative of investigative journalism (the subgenre of detective fiction in question) is being trumped in the novel and films by insisting on what Louis Marin, following Michael Fried, refers to as "the effect of seeing."[7]

"A painting of Caravaggio," Marin explains, "cannot be considered as the application of a system, or as the result (or message) of an a priori code that finds theoretical expression in the discourse on painting. The situation is quite the opposite for in producing an *effect* of 'seeing', the painting in question constitutes itself as a force, thereby distributing a series of visual effects."[8] This is how Caravaggio came to "destroy painting," in Poussin's famous phrase: Caravaggio composed canvases that, though depicting historical figures, weren't intended to recount the historical narrative but were, instead, about the act of painting itself. Hence the potency of force and impression that makes it so that one cannot tell a story about Caravaggio's paintings. Rather, the self-referentiality of representation (the fact that what Caravaggio represents in his paintings is the force of representation itself) insists on an order of mimesis that is not likeness but intensity: with Caravaggio, Marin concludes, "representation is the result of contact; vision is touch."[9]

I want to suggest that this dynamic is also at work in the movie *The Ring*. More than anything else, *The Ring* is a movie about filmic exposure that insists on a series of problems that are intrinsic to cinematic viewing. Like Marin's Caravaggio, *The Ring* is thus entirely committed to its own self-referentiality to the extent that it is committed to representing cinematic experience—and thus the effects of viewing—as an experience of dissensual immediacy.

In the preceding chapters I argued that the assumptions about conceptual artistry in the study of the history of political thought are indebted to a narratocratic regime of perception that presupposes a strict correspondence between human organoleptic arrangements and the creation of ideational artifacts. Furthermore, I suggested that such presuppositions also inform, if not define, the practices of contemporary political theorizing. To the extent that political theory is a visual practice, the movements of our eyes, mouths, and hands when reading, speaking, and writing presuppose distinct postures of attention vis-à-vis the world and others. But as we saw in the case of

Machiavelli's letter to Vettori and in our analysis of the edicola, such assumptions regarding organoleptic correspondences are, at best, questionable.

In this chapter I continue with this line of questioning by engaging the art-criticism and art-history writings of Louis Marin, Michael Fried, and Gilles Deleuze and drawing from them insights into the aesthetic and political dimensions of visuality. Specifically, I am interested in the dynamics of capture discussed by these thinkers and the relationship established between the moment of capture, the object of attention, and the viewer. My claim is that capture complicates the inherited convictions of narratocracy that sight grants us vision, and, by implication, it also complicates the relationship between viewing and narrative movement. What Marin, Fried, Deleuze, and the movie *The Ring* thus share is a commitment to understanding movement in nonrepresentational and nonallegorical terms; that is, these thinkers sustain a commitment to aesthetic experience without grounding that commitment on the telling of a story about the art object. The self-referential moment of capture in the pictorial tradition traced by Marin, Fried, and Deleuze and the conviction it engenders expose a regime of perception and the partitions that govern it.

Putting pressure on political theory's own commitment to understanding political life in narratocratic terms, I conclude that the contemporary democratic citizen-subject is a viewing subject and that the most pernicious political battles in both Europe and North America are fought at the level of audience ratings and viewership. In order to better appreciate the ethopoetic modalities of knowledge therein, it is important—if not altogether urgent—that political theorists continue to engage the regimes of perception that constitute us modern democratic subjects as viewing subjects.[10]

On Viewing and Reading

Connecting the art-history and art-theory writings of Louis Marin, Michael Fried, and Gilles Deleuze is a central problematic that might best be stated in the form of a question: how can we look at a painting and not have it tell a story? That is, how is it possible to consider an image as something other than a conduit for narrative; or, better still, how do we understand the relationship between writing and painting? Fried's own work on Thomas Eakins addresses this question directly, but I won't focus on that here.[11] Rather, my interest is in the manner in which Marin, Fried, and Deleuze, in diverse though cognate ways, engage the formal features of the visual arts by invoking visuality (or what I am calling the "effects of viewing") to distinguish between typographic representation (and, by extension, narrative and allegory) and painting. (Another way of saying this is that these thinkers draw a perceptual distinction between reading as an ocular and muscular operation of the eye that scans the page from left to right, generating a sense of narrative progress and pictorial seeing, where the muscles of the eye cannot rely on the habit of "reading movement" in order to appraise the success of an image.)[12]

In contrast to a hermeneutics of depth, these three thinkers exact a practice of viewing that emphasizes the superficiality of the canvas. Marin will go so far as to assert that "Caravaggio's gesture reveals a preference not for a depth of art but for its appearance or surface."[13] Fried's reading of Caravaggio also points to the importance of surface by directing the viewer's attention to the fact of mirror imaging in some of Caravaggio's paintings.[14] Finally Deleuze's reading of Francis Bacon insists on a mode of visual engagement that concentrates on "a single plane that is viewed at close range."[15] In all three cases, there is a theoretical commitment to not treating the visual arts as if they were similar to the literary arts. Yet at the same time, there isn't a complete elision of literariness either. Rather, the distinction that retains the tension evokes the fact that there are a multiplicity of habits of viewing that constitute an ethopoesis of the visual.

Consider in this regard Marin's treatment of what he calls *scopophilia* (the desire to see). The first thing he notes about Caravaggio is the absence of action in his paintings. Recalling *The Conversion of St. Paul* (ca. 1600) but also, ultimately, the *Medusa* shield (ca. 1598–99), Marin explains how these paintings initially present themselves as imbued with narrative—or as historical reenactments of a moment in time, whether biblical or mythological—but that they lack the kind of action that would give the narrative processional power.

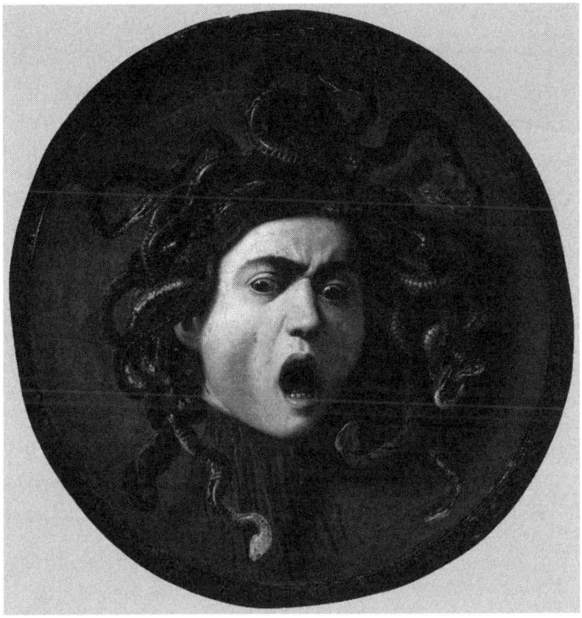

6 Caravaggio: *Medusa* (ca. 1598–99). Uffizi Gallery, Florence. Scala / Art Resource, N.Y.

In *The Conversion of St. Paul* (and also, I would say, in *The Crucifixion of St. Peter*, ca. 1600, both found in the Cerasi Chapel, in Santa Maria del Popolo, Rome), we have a kind of snapshot moment of frozen action. We may say of these paintings that they are born of a story—which is what makes them historical paintings in the first place—but these are also paintings about which no story can be told other than its title; both these paintings are committed to announcing an event (a conversion and a crucifixion) without having to recount it. Marin thus suggests that these paintings represent events without action, and it is precisely the absence of action that makes them so significant: in action's absence another force swarms in to fill the void, "the *force of painting* as a set of colors unleashing visual effects."[16]

The contrast between action and force—and, as I am implying, between reading and viewing—is one that insists on the use of color (what Marin calls Caravaggio's "color-drive") to stupefy and interrupt narrative representation. Here, the *Medusa* shield is crucial, and Marin's analysis of it is a tour de force. I won't rehearse it as it is much too detailed and intricate to recount. Suffice it to say, however, that within the trajectory that I want to establish what begs attention is the look of capture of the figures discussed. The function of color is best noted by the streaks of blood emanating from the Gorgon's neck. Like the Cerasi Chapel paintings, this too is a snapshot moment. Medusa has been decapitated, but she has also been captured, her head is in flight, but it is also mounted on a shield. In short, we have here an instant of immobility in motion when Medusa's petrifying stare is impressed as a reflection on Perseus's shield (if it weren't entirely anachronistic, one might even say "caught on tape") at exactly the moment that Perseus slays the Gorgon. The imprint on the patina of the shield is at once a representation of the moment of capture and of reflection.[17] But it is also, and crucially, a decapitation not only of Medusa but of the painter, whose painted figure is a self-portrait. "Thus," Marin asserts, "the painter inscribes himself in the painting in a dual manner, for he figures there as the petrifying and petrified gaze of Medusa, but also as the caesura of what allows him to be a gaze, namely, the head, but a head cut off at the point of its greatest power and most extreme violence."[18] And finally: "What the painting shows us and allows us to see is representation as a cut, a cutting blade severing the story from the subject who tells it while also severing the scene from those who look at it and produce it as a scene."[19]

The play on the word "execution," though never exploited by Marin, is everywhere in his account. The execution is at once the representation of Perseus's caesura and the act of painting itself; and it is this double meaning that needs to be kept in play if we are to understand the distinction between viewing and reading. For it is the interruption of the readerly repose that prevents the sensation from being reduced to mere sensationalism; or, to put this slightly differently, sensationalism results from the attempt to outline the shape—or figure—of sensation. The painting thus kills the story, as it were, precisely at the moment when it represents it, and this is why the moment of representation in Caravaggio is so stupefying: the terror of the Medusa's expression is not simply the shock of decapitation, it is also and intensely the horror of capture, the fact that she has been petrified by her own powers through the spectral play of the shield-mirror. It is the shock, in other words, of a representation that is in every respect a violence because of the caesura it executes. To say this, however, is to return to Marin's original point: "representation is not so much a distanced contemplation as a potency of effect."[20]

This potency of effect is multiplied by the fact that Caravaggio painted several scenes of decapitation (either accomplished or in the act of fulfillment): *Judith Beheading Holofernes* (ca. 1598), *Medusa* (ca. 1598–99), *The Sacrifice of Isaac* (ca. 1601–2), *Salome with the Head of the Baptist* (ca. 1609), and several *David*(s) (ca. 1609–10). There is much to appreciate in these decapitations but of particular interest are the faces of the victims or potential victims. Their mouths are exceptionally striking and, to my mind, extend the dynamics of execution theorized by Marin. In all instances, and remarkably so, the moment of shock is expressed by an open orifice, agasp in exhalation. This is the moment of life and death, when the last breath is expunged but not yet exhausted. It is, I would also say, an immersive moment (as Fried describes immersion, to which I will turn shortly). The emphasis on the face as a site of such representational potency is also significant because it imposes on the viewer a kind of physical and psychological nudity, the idea that at the moment when life encounters death, all our resources are at once exhausted and displayed on the surface. Of further note in these executed visages are the lines on the brows. In all but two (the *Salome* whose executed head is on a platter and the *David* whose Goliath was decapitated post mortem), they are tense and furrowed, as if the muscles are still contracting and, crucially, as if the face is not yet dead. To suggest that this is a liminal scene of life and death is noteworthy, but what is even more noteworthy is that these faces represent the immersive moment of shock when one's life literally flashes before one's eyes (notice also that in all these faces, the eyes are not merely glazed over—save, once again, the *Salome* and the *David*—but they look, they stare, further suggesting that though executed they are not quite dead yet).

This dynamic of life and death is extended by the fact that Caravaggio often painted the same agasp expression in many of his living faces. One need only look at the early *Boy Bitten by a Lizard* (ca. 1594) as well as the *Narcissus* (ca. 1598–99) to get an idea of the extent to which the gasping for air is at once a living moment. Indeed, it is precisely the face agasp (along with the bodily recoil in *Boy Bitten by a Lizard*) that accounts for the two representational moments that Fried discusses in his essay on Caravaggio: on the one hand, an immersive moment (linked to the problematic of absorption but not synonymous with it) of the painter caught in the "protracted, repetitive, partly automatistic act of painting" and a second moment, "notionally instantaneous, of separating or indeed recoiling from the painting itself, which is to say of no longer being immersed in the work on it but rather of *seeing* it as if for the first time."[21] (Though there is no physical recoil in the *Narcissus*, the face of Narcissus agasp staring at himself in the water also suggests the simultaneity of immersion and seeing that is made all the more palpable if we consider that his figure is literally immersed in water.) The tension between these two moments—the immersive moment of painting and the specular moment of viewing—is, I think, captured most forcefully in the tension between life and death in the agasp visages: the open-mouthed face produces the effect of shock, the indistinction of simultaneously living one's life *and* living one's death. Such a moment—which is two moments at once—generates a sense of immediacy ultimately captured in and through the decapitation paintings.

A further comparison is worth mentioning. I see the study of *St. Jerome* (ca. 1606) as expressing the same liminal features of a face gasping for breath as in these other paintings. This time, however, it is not to the living figure of St. Jerome, immersed in reading, to which we must turn but rather to the skull that sits on top of an open-faced book. The skull's mouth is also open: it is a half-skull, if you will, whose lower jaw we can't see but whose upper jaw is leaning on the open-faced book as if it were gasping for breath. The open book and the slack-jawed skull (the one signifying life, the other death) touch in their openness, as if kissing. Notice also in this painting the tension between two different immersive moments: one is Jerome reading in the right half of the painting, and the second is the

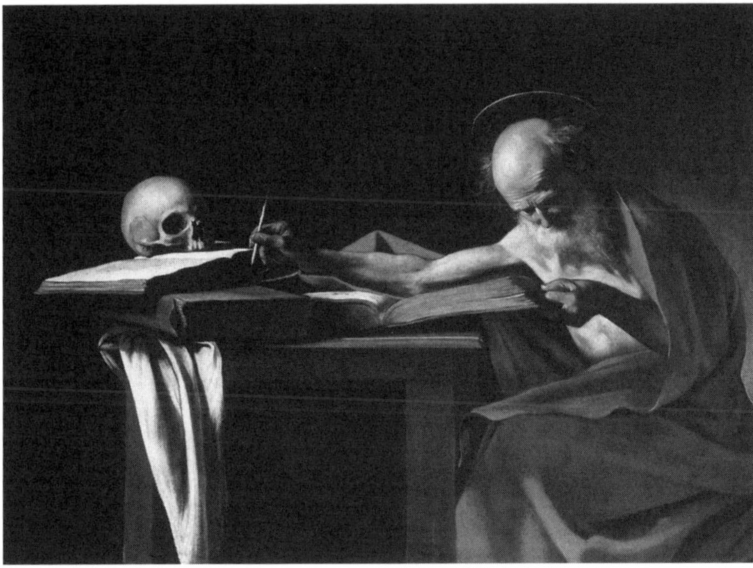

7 Caravaggio: *St. Jerome* (ca. 1606). Galleria Borghese, Rome. Scala / Art Resource, N.Y.

skull and open book as if staring at Jerome's right hand, which is holding a plume that looks conspicuously like a paint brush (or even a knife) about to execute a scene.[22] In this painting more than any other, I would say, we have an extension of the dynamics, described by Fried, in the *Boy Bitten by a Lizard*: the immersive, painterly moment (Jerome holding the plume-brush-knife) and the distanced, viewerly moment (the skull-book staring at what Jerome is holding) are geometrically parallel and simultaneous.

My insistence on the face agasp as a liminal site of life and death and as the pictorial locus of immersion and recoil is intended to extend and further emphasize Marin's and Fried's important contributions to the study of visual culture: namely, that an engagement with an art object involves an engagement with the dynamics of representation—with what Marin calls the "effects of seeing" and what I want to call, in a cinematic context, *the effects of viewing*—and not simply with the figural representations themselves or the stories that the images might or might not be telling. In other words, these critics' contribution to the study of aesthetics is to assert that the success of a work of art is not simply the result of its ability to convince mimetically, that is, through the stories that the aesthetic objects recount. Rather an engagement with the force or potency of the art object allows for the possibility of having a critical conviction without needing to revert to persuasion or belief;[23] representation, in other words, "is the result of contact, vision is touch."[24]

One final matter, by means of a transition, before proceeding to my next section: Fried's work on Caravaggio complements Marin's study and extends his own work on absorption and theatricality.[25] I want to return briefly to that work. As he explains it, absorption as theorized by Diderot is said to "somehow establish the metaphysical illusion that the beholder *does not exist*, that there is no one standing before the canvas."[26] Diderot makes this metaphysical illusion explicit in his *Salon* writings (1763–67) when he recounts with intense conviction his *promenades*. These walks are, in fact, descriptions of the paintings he is reviewing, and they rely on "the fiction of *physically entering* the painting or group of paintings . . . a fiction conspicuously at odds with the doctrine of the radical exclusion of the beholder."[27] It is, indeed, a conspicuous move by Diderot and problematic for Fried's argument regarding the parameters of absorption as a standard for aesthetic success if we interpret Diderot's fiction as one that emphasizes the viewer-beholder. But to do so, Fried explains, would be to miss a crucial point: according to that fiction, and by entering the painting and being made participant in the scene, "*the beholder is removed from the painting* just as surely as if his presence there were negated or neutralized, indeed just as surely as if he did not exist."[28]

By removing the beholder, one also removes the raconteur and, I want to suggest further, the possibility of the story of the painting as the means to justify the success of a work of art. I take this to be the point of Diderot's *repos délicieux*, the illusion that the passage of time and his very surroundings may be abolished.[29] Of course, this doesn't mean that once that aesthetic moment is accomplished, one cannot return to storytelling, as Diderot does in spades. The whole point of

Diderot's fiction of entering into the painting is that it is a fiction, a prosaic gesture he attributes to his desire to break with the monotony of description. But it is a gesture that comes after the fact, once the moment ends. At the moment of encounter with the work of art, storytelling is not an available response because the viewer is absorbed into the painting to the point that his or her status as witness is annihilated by that absorption.

We see this same moment in the works of Caravaggio, which is why Poussin accuses him of "destroying painting." To destroy painting is, of course, not to destroy the act of painting itself but rather to portray that act so intensely and so surreptitiously on the surface of the canvas, regardless of the subject being portrayed, that one can no longer say of painting, after Caravaggio, that its intent is to tell a story. Indeed, it's precisely the emphasis on the superficial space of the canvas that makes the hermeneutic depth of narrative unavailable. Caravaggio's paintings ultimately insist on the force of the surface, on the invisible sensation emanating from a thinly textured patina that impresses itself upon the senses; they insist, in the end, on rendering force by confounding the distinction between the act of representation and the subject of representation.

Rendering Forces

Gilles Deleuze's *Francis Bacon: The Logic of Sensation* begins with a chapter entitled "The Round Area, the Ring." This round area is Deleuze's way of describing the operative field that Bacon deploys to isolate the Figure in order "to avoid the *figurative, illustrative,* and *narrative* character the Figure would necessarily have if it were not isolated."[30] Isolation, in these terms, is a formal technique whereby the painter strips the Figure of any referent, forcing it to have to sustain itself. What, then, is the relevance of such an isolated Figure?

Comparable to Diderot's metaphysical illusion of entering the painting, Deleuze's insistence on the isolated Figure in Bacon emphasizes the force of sensation in aesthetic experience. "In art, and in painting as in music," he asserts, "it is not a matter of reproducing or inventing forms, but of capturing forces."[31] Bacon's paintings, like those of Caravaggio (the comparison is mine, not Deleuze's), render forces and, more to the point, make palpability a condition of viewing. Hence the function of the ring as a technique of isolation. By isolating the Figure, by radically decontextualizing it and inserting it in a denuded space where there is no presence other than the Figure itself, Bacon severs the painting from those elements that would lend it a narrative character. Bacon is thus not painting figures, nor are his paintings merely grotesque; he is, rather, making invisible forces palpable; for Deleuze, Bacon confronts the central problem of painting, the problem of rendering invisible forces.

Nowhere is this more evident than in the scream depicted in Bacon's *Study after Velazquez's Portrait of Pope Innocent X* (1953), which is so disturbing because, like Caravaggio's *Medusa*, there is no visible horror.[32] What is the scream? At one level, it is the isolated mouth. The round orifice expels horror; the open mouth is a spasm, "a movement in place."[33] We have already seen this in Caravaggio, whose open mouths are an immersive oscillation between life and death, the torsion that is at once a final exhalation and inhalation. But Bacon's mouths extend this torsion by materializing it. Whereas in Caravaggio we might easily (though I think mistakenly) slip into a mystical explanation (e.g., the soul escaping through the breath), Bacon shows us just how inappropriate such conclusions could be. The spasm is not an emerging immaterial soul, it is the intense effort of a body wanting to escape its own figure. In short, the scream is a disfiguration of the body.[34]

Here, however, we must be cautious because disfiguration is not synonymous with transformation. The disfigured body is not a resurrected body, a redeemed body about which we can tell a moving story. This is why in the 1944 triptych (*Three Studies for Figures at the Base of a Crucifixion*), two of the three figures have a ravenous mouth intent on either consumption or expulsion, but not narration. The disfigured body punctuates the effects of forces upon the body, collapsing the correspondences between the organs of perception and modes of apprehension. The disfigured body is a disorganized body, an indistinct or indeterminate body, whose only resource is sensation: "a wave flows through it and traces levels upon it; a sensation is produced when the wave encounters the Forces acting on the body, an 'affective athleticism', a screaming breath."[35]

Once we enter this zone of indistinction—where there is a disorganized body whose provisional organization endures only as long as the sensation itself[36]—we no longer possess the comfort of either narration or figuration. The horror of the scream is the horror of not having a story to tell; it is the horror that Poussin discovered in Caravaggio's works. Caravaggio destroyed painting because he painted the effects of seeing without telling stories; Bacon's scream is the spasm of a disfigured body whose modes of perception are no longer secure and whose ability to rely on sight, sound, and touch as distinct capacities is provisional to the point of evading narrative iteration. Without the assurance that our eyes grant us sight and our skin offers us touch, we can no longer assume that we know how to read and write, how to tell a story.

This, for Deleuze, explains Bacon's formula: "I wanted to paint the scream more than the horror."[37] Like Bartleby's formula discussed in chapter 1—"I would prefer not to"[38]—Bacon's formula collapses the ordered configuration of a sensible universe. The formula of deformation is a formalist intrusion that breaks the codification of formalism itself; it is a provisional aperture into a zone of indistinction that collapses the dominion of the senses. The name given to this confound is "haptic visuality."[39]

Haptic visuality, I want to argue, is Deleuze's term for what Marin refers to as the "effects of seeing" and what Fried calls "opticality." It is a term that relies on collapsing the experience of seeing and that of touching (recall Marin's claim that "vision is touch" and Fried's treatment of Diderot's "metaphysical illusion" of entering a painting), but it is also, and importantly, a mode of perception that, through visual tactility, makes narrativity insufficient to aesthetic experience. Moreover, haptic visuality compels contact with the patina of the painting; "the viewer perceives the texture as much as the objects imagined,"[40] Deleuze explains. This means, according to Laura Marks's lucid explication, that in haptic visuality the entire body is at play in a configuration and reconfiguration of sense experience. The difference, then, between haptic and ocular visuality is a matter of degree:

whereas in ocular visuality, distance matters, so that the separation between viewer and object viewed is a buffer that supports the certitude of subjectivity itself (in that one remains certain that one is a viewer viewing an object), in haptic visuality, one relies on that distance in order to collapse it, to bring the body closer to the point of (in Diderot's case) actually entering the painting. The resolution into figuration and narrative occurs only after the moment of haptic visuality, when that instant of capture has passed. An entirely provisional form of engagement, haptic visuality prevents the viewer from appreciating his or her condition because he or she is so intensely immersed in the experience of viewing that the partitions that govern his or her sensibilities no longer attain. "The haptic image," Marks rightly concludes, "forces the viewer to contemplate the image itself instead of being pulled into narrative."[41]

The confrontation with the image itself, that is, with the force of representation rather than its referent, is the important theoretical insight that Marin, Fried, and Deleuze share in varying capacities. It is a shift that I take to be crucial to the study of visual culture, and, as I will argue in my concluding remarks, an important shift in how we understand the relationship between the image, viewership, and democratic citizenship. The importance of such an approach lies in its claim that an aesthetic object ought to be engaged on its own terms, in light of its presentational properties. This doesn't mean that it is a neutral object, or that this object has no context or history. On the contrary, what this means is that in presenting itself to the viewer, the image confounds: the appearance is a singularity without model or resemblance, it is its own referent. This is the work accomplished by isolation in Bacon; the ring, round mouth, and spasm isolate the Figure and in doing so, they generate "the haunting singularity of the experiential confound."[42] And so we return to Marin's felicitous phrase, "the effects of seeing." The experiential confound is an effect of seeing that insists on the distinction between viewing and what is viewed. Within the account of aesthetic experience outlined by Marin, Fried, and Deleuze, the experience of capture results from the separation between the object and the viewing subject. When attending to the latter, we notice that the distance separating the beholder from the painting (or the viewer from the screen in the case of cinema) dissolves to the point of disrupting the distinction between the externality of the viewer and the internal frame of the object. The distance that constitutes the practice of viewing, in other words, enables its own collapse by capturing the viewer to the point of admitting him or her into the painting or screen, rendering him or her a "participant in the scene."[43]

The Phenomenology of Spooling

If (with Marin, Fried, and Deleuze) we can grasp the success of an aesthetic object without relying on storytelling, how can we understand cinematic "movement" as something other than a narrative chain of events? This question will guide us through our encounter with *The Ring*.[44] It is a question that rests on a central paradox, sustained by Jacques Rancière in *La fable cinématographique*, that the art of cinema is contrariety.[45] In *The Ring* such contrariety rests on the fact that storytelling does not break the curse of the "pestilential videotape" but that mechanic reproduction and dissemination of the film does. That is, the contrariety resides in creating a motion picture whose sense of motion is not based on plot progression but on what I will refer to as the "phenomenology of spooling." In order to appreciate this, we cannot simply rely on the story line of the movie but must also consider the effects of viewing as experienced at once in and through the movie; to invoke Marin once again, the movie in question (both the videotape in *The Ring* and the movie *The Ring*) "constitutes itself as a force, thereby distributing a series of visual effects."[46] The moment of contrariety in *The Ring* occurs when we realize that the progressive movement of our eyes reading the story from left to right (as we would a novel) is insufficient and interrupted by cinematic viewing, by the play of capture of the viewer by the screen.[47]

What, then, is "the ring"? It is the heterogeneous convergence of multiple experiential nodes:[48]

1. The ring is visual: it is the halo that forms the circle of light. It is the glare of the screen that isolates the viewer.

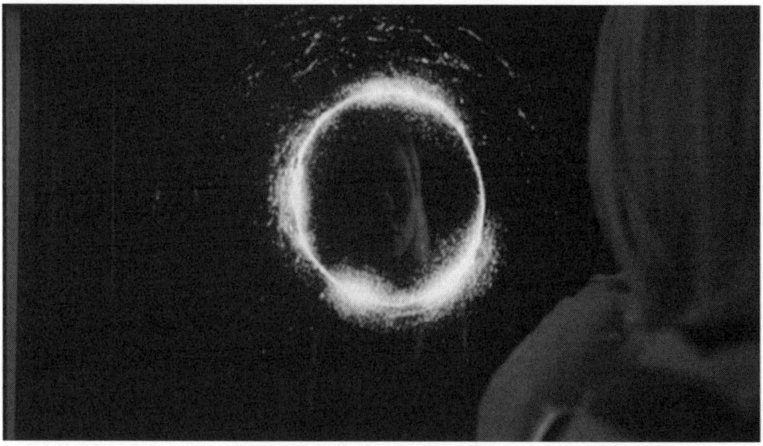

8 Rachel watching the "pestilential videotape." *The Ring* (U.S. 2002).

Immediately we are exposed to the force of viewing. Rachel (the main character in the U.S. version of the film), in a scene congruous with the absorptive pose of Diderot's *repos délicieux*, stares at a ring that captures her reflection and isolates it from the comfortable repose of figuration. Rachel is exposed to a practice of viewing—by observing the stare that is staring back at her, she is literally viewing "viewing." The moment is immersive to the point of being contagious. As in the play of capture in Caravaggio's horrified *Medusa*, Rachel is captured by the screen-eye after watching the video. Her pupils dilate and contract, and as they do, we see in them the reflection of the TV monitor as if the two convex surfaces merged so as to literally caress each other. "The ring is the last thing you see before you die," we are told over and over again in the movie. The ring's halo is thus not simply an eye, it is also the circle of light that forms around the stone covering the well where the girl is entombed. The fact that the faces of the infected victims remain imprinted with this halo represented as the open mouth (resonating affinities with both Caravaggio and Bacon—see figure 10) is thus no mere coincidence.

2. The ring is aural: it is the sound of the phone ringing, with the accompanying warning that the viewer has seven days to live.

This aural ring interrupts the moment of capture, and in so doing, it breaks the absorptive spell. It corresponds to Fried's moment of "recoil" in Caravaggio's *Boy Bitten by a Lizard*, alerting the viewer to the fact that she has been exposed to the film. But by breaking the capture, it also insists on it. Rachel clearly "snaps out of it," but by exposing herself to the impressions of the film (as the celluloid patina is itself exposed to the impressions in Samara's mind),[49] she remains contaminated and hence "captured." At this point, we can say with some confidence that the ring at once represents immersion and recoil, capture and flight, as simultaneous moments that contribute to the dynamics of conviction in cinematic viewing. The fact that after the phone rings the investigative plot gains momentum only emphasizes the tension of capture and flight. Rachel's motivation for solving the mystery is to save herself and her son from the curse. Thus, through an experiential confound that affects the eyes and the ears, Rachel experiences what Ryuji (in the novel) refers to as the "persistence of vision."[50]

3. The ring is the circle of infected viewers.

The mark of infection is imprinted onto the faces of the viewers who, when photographed after viewing the tape, are horrifically disfigured. That this mark is visible only through the photographic reproduction of the faces and that it disappears after the "pestilential videotape" is itself reproduced insists on the immediacy of the actual world and the celluloid world. After viewing the tape, in other words, the final seven days of our lives are days when we occupy both the world of the screen and the actual world, and the mark of having entered the cinematic world of the tape is disfiguration.

"The most significant thing about the photograph," asserts Deleuze, "is that it forces upon us the 'truth' of implausible and doctored images."[51] In *The Ring*, that "doctored truth" is literally stamped on the victim's faces, implausibly disfigured by the videotape's force acting upon their own bodies. And, if we wanted to extend this further and recall Deleuze's discussion of disfiguration in Bacon, we should also say that the disfigured faces represent the attempt to escape the world of the tape; they are, thus, a torsion that results from

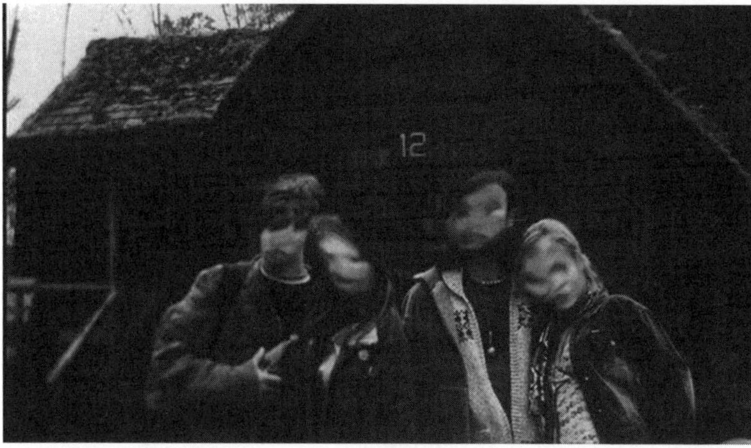

9 "Doctored photos." *The Ring* (U.S. 2002)

the intensive dynamic of capture and flight, immersion and recoil. The disfigured face marks the horrific realization that the celluloid world is a haunting parallel of the actual world to the extent that it is the real world as it appears in Samara's mind while living and dying in the well.

The disfiguration is physically accomplished once the seven days are through and the contaminated persons become victims (figure 10). The potential death that is hinted at in the doctored images is actualized by the horrible face that remains imprinted on the executed body. A visual comparison either with Caravaggio's decapitations or Bacon's "scream" hardly needs to be made other than to point out the obvious: namely, the fact that here too we have an open mouth, agasp in horror, having perhaps realized that the feeling of occupying the two worlds (the world of the image and the world of the viewer) was not merely a feeling but a reality, that there was a "truth" to the doctored image.

4. The ring is the spooling of the tape; it is succession without progress through filmic reproduction.

The phenomenology of spooling offers a repetition: the closed circularity of a film that winds and rewinds, incessantly opening itself to

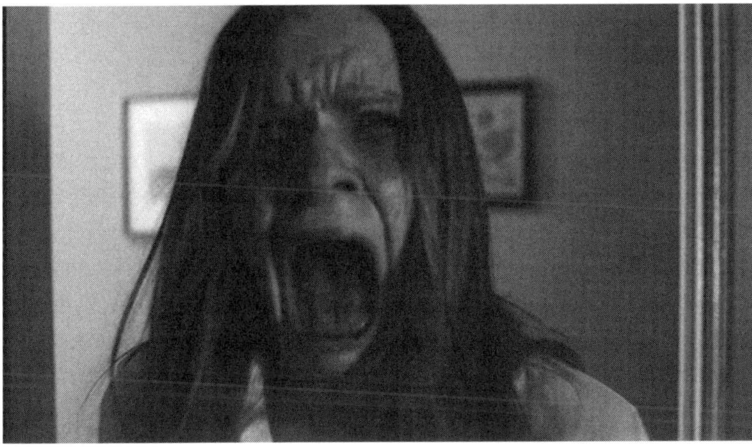

10 First victim, "Katie." *The Ring* (U.S. 2002).

projected images. This is ultimately the curse that Samara has to endure in the well, the fact that what we see on the tape are the images that repeatedly haunt her mind and that make it so that she cannot rest in peace. The repetitive spooling guarantees further contagion; an increase in ratings if you will. The continuous spooling of the celluloid strand insists on the theme of cinematic impression and production as a dominant theme of the movie. Furthermore, the circularity of spooling also implies mechanical reproduction; the reason why Samara "never stops" is because part of what constitutes the curse of the tape, like the curse of a chain letter, is the necessity of its own reproduction.

"She never stops" is the phrase pronounced by Rachel's son, Aidan, toward the end of the movie. It is a crucial line because it reveals that the movie's movement is not over, that the succession of images, contagion, projection, impression has not stopped, and neither has the movie itself. It also reveals that the allegorical reading of the movie via the plot of investigative journalism is insufficient to explain the movie and, indeed, the effects of viewing it; in short, Rachel's story has been killed because Samara's "pestilential videotape" never stops spooling. Like Bacon's scream, what is ultimately horrific about the movie *The Ring* is precisely what can be felt but not seen: namely, that redemption is not an available option if we stick to an allegorical, readerly approach to the movie. The futile attempt of trying to investigate the origin and significance of the succession of filmic images that compose what is on the videotape—that is, the attempt to convert irrational cuts into rational ones—is entirely pointless because what the tape or movie is asking from us is a cinematic mode of viewing rather than a textual mode of reading.

The Ring is about the effects of viewing to the extent that it insists on the mechanics of film (the phenomenology of spooling, the impression on celluloid patina, and so forth) but also to the extent that it insists on how this form of viewing elides, if not annihilates altogether, the presence of the viewer qua raconteur. Just as Diderot claims that the success of a work of art is to produce the metaphysical illusion that the beholder does not exist (thereby suggesting that a readerly approach to painting is insufficient), so does *The Ring* claim that the success of cinematic experience rests on haptic visuality rather than a linear, readerly visuality. The paradox, of course, is that it is only through the failure of the curative properties of narrative succession (the discovery that narrative is a snake-oil because witnessing to Samara's murder and entombment does not actually stop her curse) that we can acknowledge spooling as the movie's actual mode of motility. Once we stop reading with our eyes and start touching with our vision, we discover that the film moves along because it is being projected.

One more observation about the dynamics of visuality in *The Ring* will help me bring this discussion to a temporary close: Noah—a photographer, Rachel's past love interest, and Aidan's presumed father—is the only character in the movie whose experience of the agony of death we view. Two-thirds of the way through the movie, after we learn that Samara "never stops," we find Noah in his loft apartment and studio. Suddenly, the TV monitor flickers, and the familiar static of the white screen that we also see at the start of the pestilential tape appears. As Noah moves toward the monitor, he picks up the remote control, and in a stand-off scene reminiscent of a Western, he turns the TV off. As he walks away from the deactivated monitor, the TV turns back on, projecting an image of the well;

simultaneously the phone rings (as in the original moment of infection), but this time it is Rachel calling to warn him that the curse has not yet been extinguished. Noah does not answer because he is completely immersed in what is happening in the monitor. In the monitor we see the gradual emergence and escape of Samara from the well, making her way progressively toward the edge of the monitor and forcing herself through it in a jagged movement that mimics the visual leap we experience when skipping through a scene on a VCR or DVD player. Samara literally escapes the cornice of the monitor, as she had escaped the isolating frame of the well, and, with a force that (once again) parallels the technology of "fast-forwarding," leaps forward to face Noah. Samara's movement throws Noah back, thrashing him against a glass bookshelf. As he tries to crawl away from Samara (just as Samara had crawled her way from the television monitor into Noah's living space), she tilts her head upward, and we see her face in its post-mortem video state for the first time. The scene ends with Noah's horrified reaction, a cut to Samara's eye pupil, and a rapid succession of images that fade into the static of the monitor.

Though there is no direct correlation between Noah's death in *The Ring* and the dynamics of absorption in modernist art examined by Michael Fried, it is difficult not to acknowledge an affinity between what I have been calling the "effects of viewing" in *The Ring* and the problems related to immersion that Fried analyzes. Of a most striking nature are the affinities between *The Ring* and Courbet's *After Dinner at Ornans* (1848–49). In *The Ring* there is an attempt to overcome (or at the very least engage) what Fried celebrates as Courbet's inevitable failure: namely, "the impossibility of literal or corporeal merger that made (Courbet's) project conceivable, or rather, pursuable, in the first place."[52] That project, as Fried discusses it and as I explain above, is one of trying to defeat theatricality in painting through the absorption of the beholder into the painting so as to eliminate or elide the gap between spectator and painting, and thus remove the occasion for the experience of theatricality. This is the basis of Diderot's "metaphysical illusion," and it is, for Fried, one of the central problematics of modernist art.

The Ring accepts and celebrates Courbet's failure by inverting it: if the beholder cannot be absorbed into the work of art, and thus collapse the partition of the sensible established by the frame, then the work of art will force its way through that partition in order to enact the collapse. In both cases, however, an eradication of spectatorship occurs. In Courbet's efforts there is an implicit attempt to eliminate the beholder by absorbing her or him; in *The Ring*, the beholder or viewer is eliminated through his or her death. In both instances, and by means of extending Fried's analysis, the attempt to eliminate the viewer corresponds to the more pointed enterprise of effecting the break with the figural power of narrative. The metaphorical or metaphysical elision of the gap between object and viewer through the metaphorical or metaphysical elimination of the spectator thus crucially produces the eradication of the site of testimony and storytelling. In this manner, aesthetic experience no longer must be mediated by narrative; rather it is immediate and makes us "a participant in the scene" in the manner that Ryuji, in the novel *The Ring*, also recommends.[53]

The Viewing Subject

Haptic visuality offers us the possibility of understanding cinematic succession as something other than a narrative chain of events. In doing so it makes available a mode of cinematic engagement that acknowledges the fundamental problem of cinema as both medium and machine. By this I mean to suggest that one of the distinguishing features of cinema as a source of aesthetic experience is that it makes available film itself, the very processes by which it is at once produced and projected. By putting the "effects of viewing" on screen, *The Ring* makes what Stanley Cavell refers to as "successions of automatic world projections" palpable to the viewer.[54] This dynamic, I want to suggest finally, draws attention to the function of viewership as a practice in the modern experience of conviction. That is, by attending to the effects of viewing, *The Ring* raises a series of issues about what it means to be a viewing subject, what the regimes of perception are that we tacitly endorse in our cinematic age, and how secure we can be in our faith in a narratocratic culture of conviction; to wit, key issues for anyone living in contemporary Western democratic polities, imbued as they are by a culture of viewing.

The phenomenology of spooling that, I argue, is at the heart of the movie *The Ring* is the result of what the film theorist Gerald Mast describes as the "effective moment" in cinematic experience: the combination of its mimetic and kinetic qualities whose balance is at once variable and inconstant.[55] The ability to combine mimesis and kinesis is guaranteed by, among other things, the interplay of three types of succession: literal, imagistic, and structural. Where literal succession refers to the actual movement of filmic frames, imagistic succession points to the work of cutting that determines the length of time that an image will appear on screen, which is, ultimately, the result of the editing work of the director. Finally, structural succession refers to the film's sequence of events, what I have referred to as narrative succession.

Crucial to Mast's account of cinematic experience is the idea that in order to count as a successful piece of cinema, a film must be convincing and that the capture of conviction results from a combination of mimetic and kinetic factors characteristic of cinema (like the factors I enlist to describe what "the ring" is). In other words, the heterogeneous convergence of the succession-triptych secures conviction. To be sure, conviction here does not refer to a film's plausibility because, in that case, we could never say of a James Bond or Star Wars movie, or indeed *The Ring*, that it is convincing. The difference between plausibility and conviction resides in the ability to experience the simultaneity of the three forms of succession as successful. To leave a screening of *The Ring* and say "it didn't work for me because I don't believe in ghosts" is not a claim about one's conviction regarding the experience of the film; it is, rather, a claim about one's belief system and its relation to the sequence of events. But to make such a claim requires that we limit ourselves to only one panel of the succession-triptych; namely, structural or narrative succession. The capacity to capture, which contributes to the experience of immediacy, occurs at several levels and through the convergence of multiple organs of perception. Though it is true that a film moves steadily and successively forward, its movement is multiple; relying exclusively on plot progression to assess one's cinematic experience overshadows the interplay of other motilities that together do the work of conviction in a motion picture. Echoing Mast, we can conclude that "the appeal of the cinema is the *cumulative* kinetic hypnosis of the uninterrupted flow of film and time."[56]

The Ring's commitment to capture exploits the dynamics of conviction in cinematic experience by showing how structural succession—the chain of events—is insufficient to account for the success of that experience. The curse of the pestilential videotape is not broken once the murder is solved; rather, to break the curse one must reproduce the film and guarantee its continued literal and imagistic succession. The film's solution, in other words, comes through the dynamics of capture I have been describing: the antidote to Samara's curse lies in exploiting one's conviction to the nth degree by pirating the film so as to guarantee a fourth form of succession—transmission; it corresponds to a proselytizing imperative of conversion that says that in order to be truly convinced of one's beliefs, one must capture others and through that capture, satisfy the compulsion of having to account for one's faith.

Appeals to structural succession—to narrativity—are the basis of the commitment to vision as reading in contemporary political theory. This narratocratic commitment ultimately overlooks the kinesthetic elements that contribute to organolepsis. This, I would suggest, presents two significant problems: first, the readerly posture of attention is inattentive to the political life of sensation that resides in the dissensual moment of haptic visuality, where the tight correspondence of our modes of perception becomes, as it were, disfigured and disorganized. Second, the reliance on narrative succession as a mode of theoretical engagement is also insufficient given the condition of modern democratic citizenship: namely, that the citizen subject of modern democratic polities is not a reading subject but a viewing subject.[57]

One of the key challenges posed to contemporary democratic theory today is how to engage the image. The citizen subject is a viewing subject;[58] but viewing is not limited to mere seeing. Rather, viewing is a relay-practice at once internal and supplemental to the regimes of perception that govern visuality. There is a presumed correspondence between the eyes and seeing, hands and touching, that delimits the spatiotemporal organization of daily living. The tensions explored by Marin's, Fried's, and Deleuze's writings on painting that, I claim, are also operating in the dynamic of capture portrayed in *The Ring*, exemplify ways of disrupting a narratocratic hold on the viewer by insisting on haptic visuality as an effect of viewing.

A recent iteration of Jacques Rancière's critique of Althusser is helpful in untying the political implications of this perceptual knot. The problem with Althusser's account of the police as the petty officer, Rancière explains, is that it assumes that power resides in interpellation as if it were a kind of religious power. Rancière's "police officer," on the other hand, doesn't stop anything at all but instead insists on continuity: "'Move along! There is nothing to see here!' The police says that there is nothing to see on the road, there is nothing to do but move along. It asserts that the space of circulation is nothing other than the space of circulation."[59] Rather than relying on a mystical faith in the powers of interpellation, conviction here operates through circulation; the police officer wants us to continue to see things in the manner in which we are accustomed to seeing them, to continue to concentrate on reading at the cost of other modes of visuality. Sustaining and encouraging the circulation of things, Rancière's police officer guarantees the continuation of the organic correspondences that constitute our regimes of perception and the partitions of the sensible that make circulation possible. Moreover, by guaranteeing circulation, the petty officer also creates the self-referential possibilities of continued conviction.

The imperative that "there is nothing to see here!" and that we can rest comfortably in the knowledge that circulation is uninterrupted is, I would suggest, one of the most successful techniques of the sensible guaranteeing political conviction and allegiance. Consider in this respect William Connolly's most recent exhortations against the "evangelical-capitalist resonance machine:" "The major constituencies in the evangelical-capitalist resonance machine do not always share the same religious and economic *doctrines*. Affinities of *sen-*

sibility also connect them across links and differences in formal doctrine."[60] I would suggest that among these affinities of sensibility, these common modes of sensing, is a commitment to narratocracy that is an ennobling force in a culture of conviction so intensely rooted in reading scripture. It is not only the case that evangelical Christianity is committed to reading the Bible (as opposed to traditional Catholic doctrine that, until Vatican II, did not encourage scriptural reading for fear of heresy), it is also the case that the movement, pace, and account of sense making associated with a narratocratic regime of perception comprises the affinities of sensibility that structure the political agendas of the Children of the Book. In other words, the privilege given to narrative as the mode of political engagement coincides with an eschatological cosmology that, in turn, rests on a tight set of correspondences between organolepsis and perception (e.g., the habitual left-to-right eye movement on a page translates into an experience of historical time). It is perhaps for this reason that some political constituencies are more successful than others at the telemediatic register of citizen engagement. Aware that the citizen subject is a viewing subject, they repeatedly appeal to the narrative dimension of visual experience so as to create conditions favorable to continued conviction and circulation.

By deploying the art of cinema against itself, *The Ring* interrupts the capture of conviction and the privilege of allegorical kinesthetics. The discovery that the narrative plot in the movie is not an antidote for the curse compels us to critically assess our reliance on readerly vision, and thus reconfigure our postures of visual attention. Though the modern citizen subject may have been a reading subject, the contemporary citizen subject is a viewing subject. A critical challenge for democratic theory, then, is to engage the image; to engage the micropolitical strategies that restrict "viewing" to mere "seeing," that limit circulation to only one regime of visibility, and that insist that "there is nothing to see here!"

CHAPTER FIVE

"You're Eating Too Fast!"

Slow Food's Ethos of *Convivium*

What is known of the moral effects of different foods?

FRIEDRICH NIETZSCHE

Introduction: "Don't Speak with Your Mouth Full!"

Whereas in the previous chapter I addressed the relationship between visuality and democratic citizenship, in this chapter I explore the mouth as an organ of political reflection. Specifically, my interest is in the mouth as a complex organ of expression and consumption; in short, this is an essay about the human craving for flavor. But to write about flavor in political reflection requires that I address a normative partition: the mouth cannot eat and speak at the same time. The mouth must be either a conduit for the mind's ideas, thus making it lexically prior to all other organs in any speech situation, ideal or not. Or the mouth must be an avenue for the consumption of food, the origin of sustenance and a gustatory medium of bodily restoration.[1] In short, the mouth as organ of political reflection remains an unaddressed coefficient in the analysis of political interlocution.[2] Thus it is that our theories of justice, premised as they are on the principle of democratic deliberation or communicative action, cannot account for what Louis Marin refers to as "the ambivalence of the mouth's two spheres of orality."[3]

The possibility of separating that which makes eating possible from that which makes speech possible requires a regime of perception and a corresponding organization of the body. We may call this a priori operation by its proper name: common sense. The possibility of knowing when and how to speak, that we should or can speak at a particular moment in time, and that our words may or may not have valence (but nonetheless are sufficiently valuable that they ought to count), all these presuppositions of the proposition exist within a system of perceptual distribution that organizes an entire field of what is and is not available to sensory apprehension. The partition of the mouth as an organ for either speaking or eating is the condition of possibility for political interlocution, imposing itself with axiomatic rigor whenever we open our mouths. A first-order phenomenological principle of political philosophy, this axiom organizes and delimits an entire field of possible parts and positions. By this I mean to suggest that in order to begin to think what justice or equality are, what forms of political action are or are not legitimate, we don't simply presuppose the identity of a political subject, we also and crucially presuppose its organic makeup. The strict correspondence between organs of perception and sensory apprehension is what grants us, modern political subjects, the possibility of experiencing the phenomenality of political life. In short, we can know of the spectacle of politics because our bodies are preorganized according to the sensorial distribution of a regime of perception.

The injunction to not speak with one's mouth full that grounds the partition between speaking and eating is just such a principle of distribution. That which is used to speak and communicate one's ideas, according to our common political sense cannot, at one and the same time, count as the organ that guarantees gastronomic pleasure and bodily sustenance. Or to put it slightly differently, the mouth as a privileged organ of communication in the post-human-rights era is an independent and separate instrument from the mouth as organ of eating; and one's mode of thinking in one domain (that of free speech, for instance) ought to be separate and distinct from that in another (culinary taste). To be properly blunt, political philosophy cannot account for the confusion of associating the mouth both with the divinity of the mind and the baseness of the digestive tract.[4]

But from the perspective of the political life of sensation, the mouth is just such an ambivalent confound. Through an examination of the role of food and flavor in political reflection, in this chapter I pursue the following question: is there a taste for politics? Specifically, my concern is to explore the ethopoetic practices of convivium in the political life of sensation. I begin my inquiry by tracing the place of flavor in three canonical authors in the history of political thought: Plato, Immanuel Kant, and Jean-Jacques Rousseau. I don't linger with them too long, however. Instead, I turn to a specific taste-event in the genealogy of political flavor: the writing and publication of Pellegrino Artusi's *La scienza in cucina e l'arte di mangiar bene* (*The Science in the Kitchen and the Art of Eating Well*), first published in 1891 and recognized as the most significant Italian cookbook of modern times (by 1910, the year of Artusi's death, it had reached its fourteenth printing with fifty-two thousand copies sold). The uniqueness of this publication lies in its manner of exploiting the ambivalence of the mouth as organ of expression and consumption in order to create what the historian of food culture, Piero Camporesi, refers to as a principal text for the national unification of Italy.[5] The discussion of Artusi's role in the history of taste will serve as an introduction to an emerging and flourishing movement known as Slow Food. I conclude with an analysis of the political, aesthetic, and ethical dimensions of the ecogastronomic practices of Slow Food.

A Taste for Politics

Though rigorous in his denouncement of the senses as pertinent to the life of the mind, the most astonishing aspect of book 8 of Plato's *Republic* is the extent to which it describes the various forms of government according to their corresponding appetites. Each form has its own character, and moreover, each has its own corresponding sensorial configuration. A government of the lower orders, democracy begins when the poor take control of the reigns of power and distribute equality "to equals and unequals alike."[6] Liberty reigns therein and people are free to shop for constitutions according to their tastes, as if they were choosing fruit in a bazaar.[7] But, Plato's Socrates warns, in life there are necessary and unnecessary pleasures; necessary pleasures give sustenance and unnecessary ones are harmful. Thus, he extols,

> Will not the desire of eating, that is, of simple food and condiments, in so far as they are required for health and strength, be of the necessary class?
>
> That is what I should suppose.
>
> The pleasure of eating is necessary in two ways; it does us good and it is essential to the continuance of life?
>
> Yes.
>
> But the condiments are only necessary in so far as they are good for health?
>
> Certainly.
>
> And the desire which goes beyond this, of more delicate food, or other luxuries, which might generally be got rid of, if controlled and trained in youth, and is hurtful to the body, and hurtful to the soul in the pursuit of wisdom and virtue, may rightly be called unnecessary?
>
> Very true.[8]

The risk, of course, is that democratic peoples have no such restraint; emerging from the clutches of tyranny, the condiment of liberty will be so flavorful that they will not be capable of using it gingerly. The slippage from necessary to unnecessary pleasure, from eating to binging, is built into the character of democracy to the point that "when a democracy which is thirsting for freedom has evil cupbearers presiding over the feast, and has drunk too deeply of the strong wine of freedom, then, unless her rulers are very amenable and give a plentiful draught, she calls them to account and punishes them, and says that they are cursed oligarchs."[9] For Plato the nature of democratic life is consumptive to the point of physical and spiritual corrosion. Liberty is such an appealing condiment and has such a pleasurable flavor that overconsumption is inevitable. Democratic peoples begin by going on a shopping spree, purchasing any kind of constitution they can get their hands on according to their use and pleasure. They then proceed to luxuriate by overspicing their lives with it, and when they realize that too much is not enough, they accuse others of taking it away from them. Democratic peoples are addicts whose unrestrained sensibilities demonstrate an incapacity to govern both themselves and others.

Moreover, the desire for liberty is indistinguishable from the desire for taste, for the flavor of a condiment so powerful that it interrupts any sense of restraint. To think democratically thus means to think with and through our palates which are, ultimately, the sources of inevitable political disorder. "For Plato," Giulia Sissa explains, "the origin of disorder and the proliferation of the passions is alimentary. History captures men through their mouths. The appetite not only determines the origin of transformation, the mutation of the ideal imaginary city, but also provokes the transformation of one type of regime into another."[10] The palate is a source of sensation, of the inability to make proper judgments because of the transformation that flavor induces. Indeed, if democracy implies the dominion of equality, then it can be dissensual only to the extent that it disrupts the ordered distribution of what constitutes a proper political sense.

The flavor of freedom is as much a concern for Kant as it is for Plato. For the former, however, the experience of flavor is not as deleterious as it is for the latter. On the contrary, the arrival of taste corresponds to an experience of freedom.[11] Kant famously explains that the distinction between the pleasant, the good, and the beautiful is established by three distinct and corresponding forms of satisfaction: gratification, approval (or esteem), and that which pleases.[12] Whereas gratification concerns all irrational animals, and the approval of the good concerns every rational being (even *spirits*, Kant admits), the uniqueness of beauty lies in the fact that it concerns only humans, "animal, but still rational beings."[13] In fact, it is precisely because of the disinterested nature of a judgment of the beautiful that we experience freedom. In other words, for Kant there is no rule that forces us to have to sign on to another's reflective judgment: we are free to agree or disagree, and in doing so, we express neither our rational nor our animal natures but, indistinctly, both (see chapter 1). This means, ultimately, that a judgment of beauty can neither be grounded in an appeal to authority nor in an appeal to pleasure. The judgment of beauty, because it is uniquely free, marks a moment of dissensus: the agent of appraisal, at that moment, is neither rational nor irrational, neither animal nor human, but both. Kant then proceeds to emphasize this point by enlisting the experience of flavor: "As regards the interest of inclination in the case of the Pleasant, every one says that hunger is the best sauce, and everything that is eatable is relished by people with a healthy appetite; and thus a satisfaction of this sort shows no choice directed by taste. It is only when the want is appeased that we can distinguish which of many men has or has not taste."[14] The distinction between the pleasant and the beautiful rests on the distinction between eating because one is hungry and eating for flavor.[15] The former is bound by animal sustenance (i.e., we must satiate hunger in order to live); but the latter has no rule in that it does not follow a determinate path toward satisfaction. Indeed, in the case of taste, there is no need for satisfaction.

Both Plato and Kant are committed to flavor as a moment in the political life of sensation. This is no less the case for Jean-Jacques Rousseau. Indirectly (though probably not unwittingly) invoking Plato, Rousseau asserts in the introductory "Letter to the Republic of Geneva" of his "Discourse on the Origin of Inequality" that "liberty is like those solid and tasty foods or those full-bodied wines which are appropriate for nourishing and strengthening robust constitutions that are used to them, but which overpower, ruin or intoxicate the weak and delicate who are not suited for them."[16] The passage reads like a throwaway line that at first glance seems almost trite, given the worn metaphor. At closer inspection, however, Rousseau's literary flourish is innovative: food is a motif but Rousseau seems much more concerned with digestion and indigestion (rather than taste or flavor); and this concern, I would add, is explicitly a concern with the care of the self.

The preface to the Second Discourse that follows the "Letter to Geneva" confirms this by invoking the dictum of the Delphic oracle. But, in contrast to Thomas Hobbes's invocation of the *nosce teipsum* in the introduction to his *Leviathan*, Rousseau's turn to the care of the self is not intended as a critical attack on religious fanaticism.[17] Rather, Rousseau's invocation launches a research agenda: we will investigate how to study humans, he suggests, the "successive changes of the human constitution," "the knowledge of the real foundations of human society;" the science that brings us "a true definition of natural right . . . must be deduced from this very nature of man, from man's constitution and state."[18] And here, for the sake of brevity, we arrive at the double entendre already present in the passage from the letter: the constitution of humans and the constitution of the state. It is all too easy for us late moderns to see in these formulations the origins of modern constitutionalism—the burgeoning language of charters of rights, written testaments of "we the people," and so forth. In short, it is all too easy to see the conceptual connection that binds a Judeo-Christian heritage of covenant with the postsecular concern with contracting human rights. We should, however, resist such an easy repose of thought precisely because while Rousseau was writing the Second Discourse, this linguistic context was in coinage, though not necessarily in circulation; it wasn't part of that sense he could call common, though we can now.

The "constitution of man and state" also refers to another sense or another series of senses; for Rousseau it is a "delicate constitution" not only in the sense of a political structure but also in the potential that resides in an upset stomach as a source for political reflection: he is, in short, referring to one's physical constitution and specifically to the stomach's ability to digest things. Thus, the research project Rousseau launches in the preface and develops in the "Discourse on the Origin of Inequality" looks to a physical constitution—what humans eat and how they live—in order to assess the value of the social order. Consider, in this regard, the amount of time Rousseau spends discussing the material dimensions of the state of nature: eating, running, drinking, disease, and so forth—somatic activities that rely on an admixture of the senses. In the state of nature we do not have the advantage of having had our senses properly divided and assigned to specific organs of apprehension. Or rather, just as language has not yet been invented, neither has referentiality, nor the possibility of assigning a fixed link between word and object, sense apprehension and organ of perception.[19] For this reason he warns that "as long as we are ignorant of natural man, it is futile for us to attempt to determine the law he has received or which is best suited to his constitution."[20]

Rousseau's flirtation with a language of constitutionalism, then, begins with a discussion of digestion; that is, in his ruminations, Rousseau is intensely aware of bodily functions as sources of political thinking. Given this, we cannot overlook the extent to which both mouth and stomach are not simply organs of political reflection for Rousseau, they are also sites of political stability and instability within what Elizabeth Wingrove calls his "republican romance." In her analysis of Rousseau's *Emile*, Wingrove shows how Rousseau's republicanism is inseparable from his sexual politics as portrayed "in stories of sexual maturation that link erotic desire to doubt, violence, fear and sexual difference, and that link masculine and feminine self-awareness to the particular, material and institutional forms of interdependence and governance that characterize a republican state."[21] But sexual maturation happens later in life, and the confounding of erotic gratification and political rule that Wingrove discusses throughout her chapter on *Emile* are premised on one fundamental fact: both Emile and Sophie exist in a well-nourished state that begins with breastfeeding as the first threshold of a moral education. The second paragraph of book I begins with Rousseau's appeal to "tender, anxious mothers" and then quickly follows with this specification:

> The earliest education is most important and it undoubtedly is woman's work. If the author of nature had meant to assign it to men he would have given them milk to feed the child. Address your treatises on education to the women, for not only are they able to watch over it more closely than men, not only is their influence always predominant in education, its success concerns them more nearly, for most widows are at the mercy of their children, who show them very plainly whether their education was good or bad.[22]

More than simply a potential site of erotic desire, the mother's breast is for Rousseau a locus for the transmission of political values, and the suckling mouth is exploited for the purposes of rearing an ideal citizen, for the communication of moral sentiments, and for the nourishing of one's republican soul. "Your true republican," Rousseau reiterates in *The Government of Poland*, "is a man who imbibed love of the fatherland, which is to say love of the laws and of liberty, with his mother's milk."[23]

Distracting ourselves temporarily from textual sources, we must not overlook certain significant developments in culinary culture at the time of Rousseau's writing. The restaurant, an eighteenth-century Parisian invention, "catered not to the hungry, but to the enervated who had lost their appetites and suffered from jaded palates and weak chests."[24] Indeed, unlike the contemporary North American conception of the family restaurant, where more often than not you can have all you can eat, the origin of the restaurant was specifically a place where people went *not to eat*. Etymologically rooted in the French *restorer* (meaning to restore), the restaurant was a place where individuals of weak chests could go and consume a healthy broth, soup or other elixir without the compulsion of feeling as if they had to digest a big meal. Indeed, indigestion was a central concern of much medical know-how in the period, relying, as it did, on the interrelatedness of the digestion, circulation, and respiration triptych. "In the medical imagination of the eighteenth century, indigestion posed a constant and serious threat," explains Rebecca Spang. "According to the dominant physiological models, if one's food did not move freely through one's gastrointestinal tract, then one's blood was sure to become sluggish as well, losing its necessary liquid qualities."[25]

Restorative in the sense that it would help one's ailments, the restaurant was also able to satisfy those bland palates that were affronted by the food consumed at other eating establishments (like the inn). In this respect, frequenting a restaurant was the sociocultural marker of the aesthete, whose sensitive character was most likely to suffer the ailments of a nervous sensibility. Thus, the medical condition of being "weak of chests" was synonymous with having a nervous sensitivity: "To suffer the ill effects of digestion gone wrong was to prove the worth of one's intellectual life."[26] In this regard, there was no greater man-of-malaise than Jean-Jacques Rousseau, whose exaltation of the noble savage in the Second Discourse, along with his idealization of the simplicity of Swiss village cuisine in his best-selling *Julie, ou la nouvelle Héloïse* (1760), accompanied his own renowned delicate constitution, making him the archetype of the suffering, aesthete intellectual. Rousseau's delicate (physical) constitution became a mirror for those who sought to imitate the archetype of the sensitive soul and, moreover, was a source for his own critique of social disorder.[27] Rousseau's writings demonstrate a disgust for the social (for the corruption of the customs of modern civilization) in the same way and at the same level that his own aesthetic sensibility offered the opportunity of disgust for the overconsumption of an inn's flavorful foods. At both the physiognomic and social level, indigestion and poor circulation due to poor eating habits were to be avoided at all costs, as the final sentence of the "Discourse on the Origin of Inequality" makes clear: "it is plainly contrary to the law of nature, however defined, that children should command old men, fools wise men, and that the privileged few should gorge themselves with superfluities, while the starving multitude are in want of the bare necessities of life."[28]

That the restaurant emerged in eighteenth-century Paris around the same time as the rise in popularity of Rousseau's delicate constitution is no surprise according to Rebecca Spang. The restaurant is a cultural locus of a series of convergences of political, aesthetic, physiognomic, and culinary sensitivities. A delicacy of taste, guaranteed by a public display of private sensitivity through the sipping of a consommé at an intimate table, made it possible for people to witness each other's tastes and, in the same regard, to attest to the delicacy of one's mouth and stomach as organs of political reflection.

Though it may be true, as Eric Schlosser notes in his best-selling *Fast Food Nation*, that "the human craving for flavor has been a largely unacknowledged and unexamined force in history," it is also true that this craving is consistently enlisted by writers in the history of political thought.[29] My discussion has thus far focused on the centrality of the mouth as a complex organ of political reflection. Its complexity lies in the fact that the mouth is at once an organ of transmission for the mind's ideas and an organ of consumption for the body's sustenance. Scholarly attention, however, has focused almost exclusively on the mouth as the medium of speech, thus overlooking the myriad of cultural and political possibilities in the mouth's pursuits of flavor. The theoretical point that accompanies this interjection is that whenever appeals (whether metaphorical or otherwise) are made to the mouth and flavor, as we see with Plato, Kant, and Rousseau, there is an implicit acknowledgment of a confounding of our perceptive competencies that accompanies the political life of sensation. The complexity of the mouth as an organ of political reflection carries with it a potential disarticulation of the correspondences presupposed by our organs of perception: all of a sudden, perception becomes a problem (as Merleau-Ponty might say), a new configuration of sensation is introduced, and with it a new posture of attention.

The Art of Eating Well

Roland Barthes's brilliant explication of the Panzani billboard in "The Rhetoric of the Image" presents an image of Italianicity that is easily recognizable given the proliferation of "*hospitaliano*" eateries in the world. Indeed, as a representative of Barilla recently explained at the inaugural symposium of the ALMA international cooking academy in Colorno, Italy, one of the most difficult things that Barilla had to overcome when accessing foreign markets was precisely the *image* of Italianicity.[30] The partitions of the sensible were rigorous: it was imperative for Barilla to justify to consumers that just because something looked like pasta that did not mean that it was pasta;[31] the play of denotation and connotation that organizes Barthes's reading of the Panzani billboard, though helpful at the level of advertising, was also the obstacle at the level of market shares. Here the difficulty arose in explaining the superior value of durum wheat pasta in its ability to both retain texture and combine with the flavor of the pasta condiments. Durum wheat pasta is unique in its capacity to keep the "al dente" texture after it is cooked, all the while releasing the appropriate amount of starch that fuses with the pasta condiment.[32] In the Panzani billboard imaginary, if it looks like pasta, it is pasta regardless of its "al dente" potential.[33] The point of the Colorno ALMA academy and Barilla's intervention in the preparation of pasta was to insist on the importance of flavor and the education of taste in an era dominated by the industrialization of food.[34]

To be frank, the possibility of engaging the Panzani billboard in the manner that Barthes recommends relies on an assumption about Italy that is a very recent invention, given the peninsula's history of appetite:[35] namely, the idea of plenty. The "vita" of Italian food consumption from unification in the late nineteenth century to today was not as "dolce" as the post–Second-World-War Fellini images have made it out to be. Indeed, as Carol Helstosky has shown, "the most immediate and visceral element" unifying Italians after the Risorgimento and well into the twentieth century was a poor diet. It wasn't simply the case that meat was a rarity; white bread or pasta rarely appeared on Italian tables either, and polenta and potatoes were the main source of sustenance.[36] Moreover, it was as the result of Italian immigration to the Americas in the 1920s that food industries like dried pasta, canned tomatoes, and olive oil were able to develop. "Ironically, it was because of the 'imagined communities' outside Italy that the food industry inside Italy produced the goods that became the foundation of Italian cuisine."[37] Italian immigrants who were able to make more than a subsistence income in North and South America could afford to purchase prepackaged dried pasta made of expensive grains, and since by 1920 about one quarter of the Italian population had left the country, this meant that there was a burgeoning market that could sustain the industrial production of food. Thus, Helstosky concludes, scarcity and not abundance shaped the national cuisine of Italy.

Whereas scarcity unified the Italian nation through the pursuit of the satisfaction of hunger, Pellegrino Artusi's publication of *La scienza in cucina e l'arte di mangiar bene* (1891) contributed to national unification by appealing to the palate. "The Artusi"—as it is referred to in every Italian home to this day—was the first cookbook for the household; moreover, it was the first cookbook to meticulously collect the culinary rules and advice for the preparation of traditional foods and flavors found throughout Italy. But the reader of the Artusi should be forewarned: though its imaginary is Italy writ large, Artusi is clearly taken by the Parma-Bologna-Firenze triangle. Its linguistic style is Florentine and its culinary emphasis is Emiliano. Moreover, when reading the Artusi, one cannot overlook its class imaginary: appeals to the emerging (or struggling to emerge) bourgeoisie are everywhere, not the least in the title itself: the vision of science and the constant suggestions for hygienic handling were part and parcel of a bourgeois vision of good cooking. Also relevant are its anti-Gaulic sentiments that further betray Artusi's commitment to unification. Italy is no longer part of France, and French cooking needs to be purged, as the following recipe for codfish suggests:

> 118. Baccalà Montebianco (Salted Codfish Mont Blanc Style)
>
> How strange is the nomenclature associated with cuisine! Why white mountain and not yellow mountain, as one would think from the color this dish takes when made? And how could the French, demonstrating their usual boldness when it comes to metaphors, have stretched their name for this dish into *Brandade de morue*? *Brandade*, they say, derives from *brandir*, to move, strike, wave a sword, halberd, lance and similar weapons. In fact, what is being brandished except a paltry wooden mixing spoon? No, it cannot be denied that the French are clever in everything!
>
> Whatever the case, this is a dish that deserves your full attention, because salted codfish, when prepared in this fashion, loses its vulgar nature, becoming very delicate and gracing an elegant table, either as an appetizer or *entremets*.[38]

Unforgiving and relentless in his attack, Artusi begins his description of this traditional Provençal dish with concern over its name and, implicitly, over the French inability to distinguish between white and yellow. Artusi is being particularly acute in his criticism, given that the dish most likely originates from an area near Mont Blanc. But precisely because of his desire to reterritorialize the dish, he implies that the adjective "blanc" is a misnomer since the color of the dish—due to the addition of olive oil to the cream—makes it yellow. Artusi never tells us, however, whether the original recipe adds olive oil to the cream or uses butter instead, as is more traditional in French cooking. If it did use butter, then the dish would look more white than yellow. But this is speculation on my part; what is certain is that in his account Artusi does not even mention the geographic association with Mont Blanc. Rather, he derides the French name for the dish, suggesting that their capacity to create such pretentious metaphors is an instance of clever catachresis: there is no brandishing of a "big sword," Artusi extols, there is merely a loose-wristed swinging of a "paltry wooden mixing spoon." For an Italian audience of the late nineteenth century, the sexual innuendo is unimpeachable, and the emasculation of the French in the kitchen and battlefield is just one of the many political commentaries that exemplify Artusi's wit and ability to conquer popular appeal through words and palate.

More than anything else, the Artusi is an instance in the genealogy of the mouth-confound. Though written in an appealing style, one cannot limit an appreciation of its documented appeal (and indeed, the success of the publication) to its linguistic acumen: it is appealing, I would further suggest, because it repeatedly insists on the queer connection between the names of dishes, the proper names to give recipes, and the specific value of their flavor. It is as if Artusi is suggesting that in order to know why a recipe should be called what it is, it needs to be tasted. The referentiality of naming, in other words, is grounded on the delicacy of taste:

> 455. Cacciucco I (Fish Stew I)
>
> Cacciucco! Let me say just a little bit about this word, which is understood perhaps only in Tuscany and on the shores of the Mediterranean, since on the shores of the Adriatic it is called "brodetto." In Florence, "brodetto" means a soup with bread and broth, bound with beaten eggs and lemon juice. In Italy the confusion between these and other names from province to province is such that it is almost a second Tower of Babel.
>
> After the unification of Italy, it seemed logical to me that we should think about unifying the spoken language, and yet few can be bothered with such an undertaking and many are outright hostile to it, perhaps because of false pride and the ingrained habit the Italians have of speaking their own regional dialect.[39]

Perhaps the resistance is not so much due to the false pride of Italians as to Artusi's own hubris in assuming that the unifying language should be a Florentine Italian—a contested assumption in Italy since Dante's time. Be that as it may, the concern over naming is peppered throughout Artusi's magnum opus; but rather than in the mind, these language games play themselves out on the palate. "Taste cacciucco," he is saying to his readers, "and then you will know why the Florentines have named it correctly." To call it "brodetto" as they do on the other side of the peninsula is a misnomer simply because brodetto means soup and not "stew," which is what cacciucco is.

To focus our attention on the potential of an essentialist ontology in the Cacciucco recipe or, perhaps, condemn Artusi for his appeals to elegance and delicacy in the Baccalà Montebianco recipe (with its final appeal to the restoration of codfish from a vulgar dish to one worthy of an elegant table) would only be possible if we were to overlook the fact that, within the context of a gastronomic culture of scarcity, Artusi made these tastes available to a multitude of people who had never had access to them. Artusi's is, as Piero Camporesi has rightly asserted, "a divulgated and democratized cuisine of the nobles."[40] Released from their exclusivity, these recipes entered the popular Italian imaginary, popularizing a delicate palate regardless of the frequency with which the recipes could be served. In short, Artusi is not writing for a noble readership or for the aristocrat whose privilege defines his or her capacity for taste; a foreign founder, he inverts this assumption—as Kant had in his *Critique of Judgment*—by affirming that one does not require either rank or status in order to acquire a refined palate.[41]

Artusi, I want to suggest finally, is the kind of foreign founder that Bonnie Honig discusses in her *Democracy and the Foreigner*: he self-consciously attempts to articulate "an alien experience, giving it cultural organization while also displacing it outward."[42] In contrast to Honig's symbolic reading of foreign founding, however, I am suggesting that the success of Artusi's foreign founding is in his ability to confound the senses by making available disparate flavors to groups and individuals that would not have had the opportunity to experience them previously. Italy, though territorially unified, did not exist as a national consciousness (some say it still doesn't). Artusi's plan for unification seems relatively effective in that regard: by appealing to the complexity of pleasure through the mediation of the science-practice-art triad of a post-Kantian modernity (that plays out through his commitment to hygiene, economy, and good taste),[43] Artusi thought himself capable of generating palatable lines of attachment by appealing to the pluralization of the particularity of taste. Unification for this foreign founder did not mean the subsumption of the diversity of flavors under a general, common sensory experience. On the contrary, unification was possible only through the celebration of particularities because this, more than anything else, was the only common cultural principle that the disparate regions of the peninsula shared: a general pleasure in the particular. In so doing Artusi is able to challenge the comfort with which we rely on reading as a principal mode of political reflection through his appeals to taste and through the incessant array of centripetal and centrifugal forces that compel the reader and cook to experience the particularity of a dish's flavor on his or her own palate in order to be persuaded by the linguistic claims Artusi makes. Artusi's *La scienza in cucina e l'arte di mangiar bene* is an organoleptic document of the political life of sensation based on the pleasures of the art of eating well.

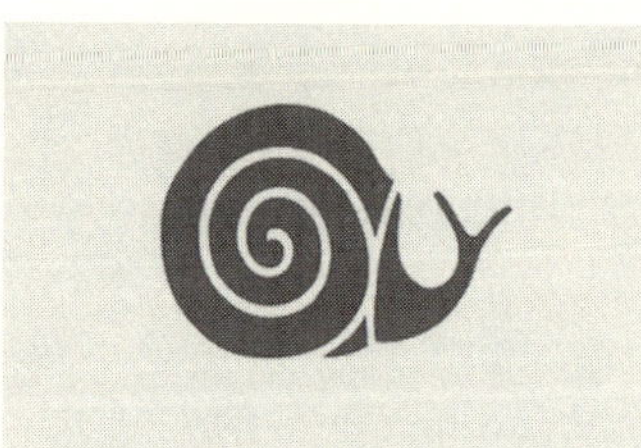

11 Slow Food logo *(with permission).*

By the second half of the twentieth century, once the prosperity of the Marshall Plan guaranteed Italy the possibility of an increased standard of living, the patterns of food consumption began to change. The construction of canteens, cafeterias, and bars or caffè's, as well as the collective feedings which took place in those institutions, made it so that Italians no longer had to concern themselves with filling their stomachs. Moreover, though the relationship between food and party politics was nothing new, after 1945, the Christian Democratic Party promoted its ability to put food on Italian tables, with the assistance of the United States. A poster from the infamous 1948 contest between Christian Democrat Alcide De Gasperi and Communist Palmiro Togliatti made the campaign stakes perfectly clear: "Don't think that with Togliatti's speeches you'll be able to flavour your *pastasciutta*. All intelligent people will vote for De Gasperi because he's obtained free from America the flour for your spaghetti as well as the sauce to go with it."[44] The advent of the Italian republic saw the cold war played out on the mouths and in the stomachs of voters. The *Festa dell'unità*—the Italian Communist party's yearly traveling festival—along with the plethora of public food festivals called *sagre* all feature eating as a principal marker of citizenship.

Postwar industrialization also brought with it changes in social structures and patterns of living that are, by now, predictable features of globalization: a shift in dwelling patterns from the extended to the nuclear family, a mass migration to the cities from the rural areas, the progressive elimination of the interrupted work day in favor of the North American model of the continuous work day, and so forth. With the increase in consumer spending came a paradoxical decrease in attention to the pleasure of the particular. The process described by Eric Schlosser—of "the Chicken McNugget turn[ing] a bird that once had to be carved at a table into something that could easily be eaten behind the wheel of a car"[45]—started to take hold in the 1980s and came to a clash on March 22, 1986 when the McDonald's corporation tried to open one of its restaurants in Piazza di Spagna, Rome. That day saw massive protests, and though the protests were not successful in suppressing the opening of the McDonald's, they were successful in changing its architectural appearance. It is this day that, for all intents and purposes, marks the beginning of the Slow Food movement.[46]

The ebbs and flows of the movement had begun prior to that day. Its founder and architect, Carlo Petrini, was already working in his native region of the town of Bra (in Piemonte) in the 1970s with a politically left cultural activist movement called ARCI (Associazione

Ricreativa Culturale Italiana). In the early 1980s Petrini became involved with the development of the Langhe Barolo wine, close to Bra, through the Free and Praiseworthy Association of the Friends of the Barolo. This commitment to local associations and their indigenous products is, for Petrini, supported by his readings of the early nineteenth-century thinker Brillat-Savarin whose *Physiology of Taste* (1825) expounds on a materialist philosophy rooted in gastronomic culture.[47]

The November 3, 1987 issue of *Il gambero rosso* ("The Red Shrimp," the cooking insert of the left-wing Italian newspaper, *Il manifesto*) published "The Slow Food Manifesto." Eventually approved and adopted by delegates from sixteen countries at the *International Slow Food Movement for the Defense and Right to Pleasure* symposium in Paris (November 9, 1989), it announced that the twentieth century was the century that took the machine as its life model and declared modern humans to be "enslaved by speed." "To be worthy of the name," it proclaims, "*Homo Sapiens* should rid himself of speed before it reduces him to a species in danger of extinction. A firm defense of quiet material pleasure is the only way to oppose the universal folly of the Fast Life."[48] To be sure, the "universal folly of the Fast Life" should not be grasped simply: that is, as a Luddite attack against the notion that an accelerated tempo of life eliminates the pace appropriate to democracy. After all, there is much material pleasure in driving fast, or allowing oneself to be captured by the force of gravity when diving into crystal clear water. Slow Food's commitment to "slow," rather, is at once a rejection of the idea that only one temporality is acceptable to modern living and an acknowledgment of the importance of the asymmetries of pace that encourage democratic pluralization and foster its fragility.[49] The "universal folly of Fast Life" is just that: foolish because universalist in its application.

Under the banner of the snail, Slow Food recommends a return to the table.[50] The table is the cultural object that represents the transversalism residing in the movement's commitment to an ethos of *convivium*. The symbolic status of the table is a well-established metaphor in theories of political communication, as Romand Coles has argued.[51] Coles's turn toward a conception of tabling "that moves and transforms but does not vanish"[52]—the radical democratic table —is helpful in demonstrating the extent to which those agreements reached through the act of tabling continue to shape and alter our lives. Yet, this is still a communicative table like the table in a board room or a seminar; Coles's table is a talking table where actions are justified, decisions are made, sides are taken; engaging only one dimension of the mouth, one cannot eat at this table because it is intended for speaking.

From the perspective of a transversal ethos of convivium, the table is much more than a conduit for communication; it is a source of material pleasure that may include speaking but is certainly not reducible to it. The communicative table, in other words, is inattentive to sensation to the extent that its purpose comes into being when perceptual divisions are already in place. The table of convivium is transversal to the extent that it comes into existence not through a presanctioned regime of perception but, rather, through its collapse and reconstitution at the moment of gustatory impact, through the overlapping of flavors and the heterogeneous convergence of both natural and human factors that contribute to the particularity of taste. Transversalism, then, differs substantially from cosmopolitanism: not committed to cosmopolitanism's various deliberative and distributive assumptions about sensory convergence, convivium understands the table as a site for the interruption of the commonality of sense. Privileging the pluralization of particularities, it endorses a variety of concrete practices rooted in the pleasures that emerge from the art of eating well.

Slow Food espouses four fundamental principles: the first is a continued attention to the study of material culture by learning how regional foods are produced; second, to preserve agricultural and alimentary heritage from environmental degradation. Here, again, the emphasis is on taste and what Petrini calls "the organoleptic profile of the food we eat (how it strikes our sensory organs)."[53] Third: to inform the producer and consumer where to find the right combination of quality and price, "neither praising things that are good but expensive nor those that are cheap and substandard."[54] And finally, "to research and promote the pleasures of gastronomy and conviviality, in a congenial and tolerant manner that encourages an approach to food based on the hedonistic advantages of deeper knowledge, the education of the senses, and harmony around the table."[55]

As idealist as this procedural apparatus may seem, it is based on concrete principles of human interaction. The first of these is a generosity and respect for the human environment: the individual of convivium is, not surprisingly, convivial; "she is jovial and optimistic by nature and is able to communicate these qualities in daily life, and especially at meals."[56] This individual is also not intimidated by pleasure. This is not to say that she is an obsessed consumer; on the contrary, to consume and to enjoy are two distinct and separate activities. The former dulls the capacity for taste while the latter develops it. "If hamburgers are being consumed mechanically and giving the same stimulus again and again to the sense organs of the young," Petrini explains, "then we have to undertake a campaign of permanent education of the taste buds."[57] Part of this education involves the development of attentiveness to the selection of ingredients and, most notably, to the pleasure of flavors.

The capacity to experience something attentively is extolled at the table of convivium. Rather than being anxious about putting one's ideas out "on the table" and marking them with quick-witted punctuality, an ethos of convivium endorses the taking of time to not only enjoy what is available for sensory experience but to learn how to be attentive to that experience, aware of when it might begin and end, how it tastes, and most notably, the ambiguities experienced at the intersections of flavors. Slow Food's commitment to slowness has nothing to do with a romantic reappraisal of pastoral life, nor is it an embrace of the terrapin time of nostalgia and tradition.[58] On the contrary, "slow" marks a durational intensity that involves appreciating the measures of time, the multiple temporalities of human life that transverse the diurnal living of individual beings. In short, "slow" refers to the practice of a political part-taking of time. In a global political economy governed by the pursuit of profit without pleasure, Slow Food enlists the pursuit of pleasure in order to interrupt the speed of profit.

This particularist ethos also informs the movement's ecogastronomic practices.[59] Biodiversity, Petrini argues, is the first step toward the enjoyment of particularized pleasures. In 1997, following a rise in the movement's international appeal, organizers formed the Ark of Taste—a conservationist practice (based on the "Noah principle") that attempts to address the problems outlined in the Slow Food Manifesto by locating and encouraging the purveyors and growers of fine foods and protecting them from the pressures of the industrialization of flavor. To be sure, the Ark of Taste is not a museum; it is a *presidium* that has saved over two hundred species of foods from extinction including the Malaysian adan buda rice grain, Moroccan argan oil, Polish Oscypek cheese, and the UK's artisan Somerset cheddar.

From the Latin meaning "armed garrison," the presidium is also responsible for the protection of the Bourbon Red and Narragansett American turkeys. Most turkeys traditionally consumed at Thanksgiving and Christmas are of the Broad-Breasted White variety (BBW), a beast that "has been so thoroughly industrialized that it can no longer fly, survive outdoors, or reproduce without help."[60] The Bourbon Red and Narragansett, unlike the BBW, do not guarantee the plumpness at Thanksgiving associated with a Norman Rockwell imaginary of the feast. Furthermore, because they actually use their legs, these heritage birds need to be cooked in a different manner than simply putting them in a convex oven for four hours. However, as *Mother Jones*'s Michael Pollan confesses after attentively preparing a Narragansett for Thanksgiving, "simply by virtue of having flavor, this represented a completely different order of turkey. Now I understand what turkey was like before the advent of the Broad Breasted White, and why turkey had once been considered a great treat."[61] It was neither through the turkey's presentation nor its size that the culinary event of "tasting the turkey" occurred, but rather on the palate and through its flavor. The tasting of turkey alerted Pollan as to why such a conventional bird, which is usually experienced as a cold-cut loaf, had been such a treat (in other words, taste actually provided pleasure). The organoleptic experience of a Narragansett turkey also helped them grasp why turkeys were important to Thanksgiving and, I would argue, assisted in the ethical affirmation of gratitude. Pollan and his friends at the table were ultimately grateful for the treat, for the pleasure they shared in their own convivium.

The convivium does not simply connote the transversal ethos of Slow Food; it is also the name of international, local structures that are the backbone of the movement. Small groups headed by a democratically chosen "fiduciary," these convivia organize gastronomic events and discussion forums that constitute "a geographical mosaic with multiple intersections, where borderlines are traced by a change in the ingredients of a *sugo* (sauce), a different method of cooking, the presence in the fields and orchards of a certain grape variety or vegetable or fruit."[62] In these instances, the development of the capacity to make distinctions is imperative; but, Petrini insists, it is not intellectual distinctions that need to be made. Rather a transversalist ethos of convivium attends to the primacy of sensory experience, relying on the senses to discern the quality of material life, including the materiality of human interaction. Like Artusi, Petrini also acknowledges our palates as the loci of an ethical battle of geopolitical proportions. Taste, in other words, is a source of ethical life, and our abilities to extricate our palates from the standardization of a globalized gastronomy—epitomized in one of McDonald's corporate slogans, "One taste world wide"—reside in the potential found in the transversalist principle of an ethos of convivium: pluralize your mouth and savor the pluralization of particularities.

Convivum, Transversalism, and the Care of the Self

Here is what I mean by a principle of transversalism that accompanies an ethos of convivium: transversalism is a cutting-across movement over thin surfaces that lack the capacity and thickness to anchor. A transversal implies an intersecting system of forces like a beam of light, a muscle, a wave; it implies the fluctuation of intensities that pulsate in and through one another as does the pungency of a spice, the spasm of indigestion, the torsion of a cramp. A transversal principle of an ethos of convivium is imbued with sensation, but there is nothing that dictates its form, shape, or motion. Because it is transversal and convivial at the same time, it is at once dissociative and associative, ebbing and flowing between detachment and attachment. It refers, in brief, to a dissensual *living with* the world and the taste encounters it affords: at one level, a transversal ethos of convivium dissents from the apodicticity of a cosmopolitan aesthetic that praises the continuity of flavor (to wit, a common sense). But it is also dissensual in that it refuses to be persuaded by the conventional confidence that our current organoleptic arrangements are as they must be, unalterable and necessary.

The dissensual delight of an ethos of convivium points to a concrete discord of the faculties: consider, once again, Michael Pollan's discovery of the flavor of the Narragansett turkey. This experience was not simply pleasant, it disfigured Pollan's sensorial capacities, thus reconfiguring his experience of what it means to taste flavor and, ultimately, his historical and contemporary intuitions about gratitude: to mark gratitude by eating turkey in a Pilgrim culture theologically resistant to the extravagances of taste must have meant a commitment to flavor as part of a community-constituting experience. The Pilgrims, in other words, were as grateful for the flavor of the bird as they were for the bounty it symbolized. Had Pollan's experience of taste been limited only to a rethinking of what counts as "good turkey," that would have been sufficient to justify the arduousness that he and the cultivators of the Narragansett bird went through in order to present it on the table. But Pollan's experience is much greater than this: through the disarticulation of visual and culinary organolepsis, there is a rearticulation of pleasure, a rearticulation of the conviviality of sitting at a table, and a rearticulation of gratitude. The bird, because less plump, did a disservice to the Norman Rockwell image of what a proper Thanksgiving dinner ought to look like. But the interruption of that image through the pleasure of taste reconfigured Pollan's ethical imaginary: now he better appreciates the gift of thanks and is himself grateful for flavor. This moment of savory dissensuality puts a new twist on the idea of comfort-food: there is, I suspect, nothing comforting in the exuberance of flavor that comes with the eating of the Narragansett bird. On the contrary, what we have here is the disfiguration of comfort through an encounter with taste.

In the introduction to this book, I suggested that our understandings of common sense are carriers of a regime of perception and a corresponding conception of the organic makeup of our bodies. Thus, we feel confident when we assume that our eyes assist sight, our ears sound, our hands touch, our noses smell and our mouths taste. But the confidence in such correspondences relies on an inattentiveness to sensation and, specifically in the case of flavor, to an inattentiveness to the complexity and ambivalence of the mouth as an organ of political reflection. From Plato through Kant, Rousseau, and Artusi to Slow Food's commitment to a transversal ethos of convivium, we notice how the mouth, rather than guaranteeing the knowledge and continuity of habitual sense, confounds. The result is a disfiguration of the body's organic constitution that corresponds to a form of life Deleuze describes as "the Body-without-Organs."

The political life of sensation does not assume that bodies are pre-organized. Rather, they are continually constituted and reconstituted through encounters with external forces: paradoxically, organolepsis disorganizes the body. When a food particle enters the mouth, a sensation occurs that configures an organ of perception which, in turn, lasts as long as the sensation, only to be displaced and posited elsewhere. The flavor sensation at once articulates the domain of its organ and disarticulates the regime of perception that had previously existed: "The BWO [Body-without-Organs] is opposed not to the organs but to that organization of the organs called the organism . . . the organic organization of the organs,"[63] Deleuze explains. He adds, "the organism is a phenomenon of accumulation, coagulation, and sedimentation that, in order to extract useful labor from the BWO, imposes upon it forms, functions, bonds, dominant and hierarchized organizations, organized transcendences."[64]

That the organism's purpose is to extract useful labor grants us purchase into what might otherwise be an obscure political metaphysic. The figure of the organism in Deleuze corresponds to the conception of common sense: its task is to organize, to impose form, and to delimit the movement of flows; it is able to extract useful labor because it can decide which organized forms of living are, in fact, most productive. The figure of the organism is at the heart of the logic of generality that an ethos of convivium, by privileging the pluralization of particularities, is committed to disrupting. The organism, in other words, is what is presupposed in a theory of sense inattentive to sensation. Relying on the correspondences guaranteed by a presupposed regime of perception, the function of the organism is to make sure that things flow and that circulation is uninterrupted. But sensation interrupts sense, flavor unravels organolepsis. Plato, Kant, and especially Rousseau were intensely aware of this, as were Artusi and, today, the members of Slow Food.

Beyond emphasizing the role of the political life of sensation, there is another dimension to the Body-without-Organs that is relevant to our discussion of taste.[65] Recall how Kant reconfigures our pleasure synapses by insisting that there can be no rules to impose a judgment of beauty. Beauty is disinterested and hence egalitarian precisely because it cannot be motivated by a normative apparatus. Thus, only taste can guarantee the experience of freedom equally and by anyone. For Deleuze to claim that "the BWO is opposed not to the organs but to that organization of the organs called the organism" is to assert exactly the same Kantian aesthetic principle at the level of sensation: just as for Kant there exists no faculty that possesses the authority to legislate taste, so for Deleuze no one organ of perception has the authority to legislate sensation.[66] What does this mean? Simply put, this means that, in human affairs, politics, and life more generally, there is no process of justification that guarantees the perceptual privilege of the eyes over the mouth, the nose over the ears, and so forth. For both Kant and Deleuze it means that there can be no regulative ideal and no a priori regime of perception adequate to explain and justify value.

"One ought not to speak and eat at the same time," Louis Marin explains, "for fear that an always possible short-circuiting might occur. For fear that the two functions, both of which take place between the lips and the throat, might suddenly be inverted."[67] In the preceding pages, I explore the short-circuiting of the mouth-confound through an analysis of flavor and the transversal ethos of convivium. I explain how such an approach attends to the political life of sensation and the means by which individuals constitute themselves as subjects of perception through such practices as eating, tasting, viewing, and reading. Sensation, as we have seen, is an experience that does not rely on a given form of sense making; it is, in all respects, dissensual. And yet, despite its indistinction and indeterminacy, it is nonetheless crucial to political life.

It is, I would add, crucial to ethical life also. Our encounter with Artusi's oeuvre shows this. His ethical imperative is not categorical but worth considering nonetheless: "know how to rule well your stomach, how to have dominion over your self." It is a not so subtle extension of what Foucault, one century later, developed as a hermeneutics of the subject.[68] Artusi, in other words, is entirely ensconced in an ethopoesis of the self that, ceteris paribus, is at the heart of Slow Food's commitment to an ethos of convivium. By proclaiming the need to relearn how to taste and by defending a right to pleasure, Slow Food adopts a commitment to un-learning (*de-discerere*); the first step, Foucault explains, in the care of the self. Like the consommé of the eighteenth-century restaurant, this form of care is restorative in its therapeutic orientation: we work on our palates in order to transverse the set of flavor relations to which we have become accustomed, so as to have the kind of care for ourselves that will, in turn, allow us to care for others. Biodiversity and ecogastronomy begin with the refinement of the palate, with the breaking of our gustatory habits and a rediscovery of the pleasures of sensation that Plato so admirably affiliated with democratic life.

EPILOGUE

"The Photographs Tell It All"

On an Ethics of Appearance

> The world is a mobile texture of these distinctions between seen and seeing objects. It is the stuff in which the inner folding, unfolding and refolding takes place which makes vision possible between things. MICHEL DE CERTEAU

In the spring of 2004, as I began researching some of the material in this book, I was invited to give a public lecture at the Nuova Accademia di Belle Arti (Santa Giulia) in Brescia, Italy. I gladly accepted the invitation as it was my first occasion to speak with an audience of artists, architects, and their students. As convivial as the event turned out to be, I was struck, during the question and answer period, by the audience's insistence on the intensity and presence of some of the images I had projected during my talk; a force, I gathered, that seemed unrelated to their interpretive horizon or context. The images were neither controversial nor dramatic but mostly of the illustrative variety (I had recently learned how to use PowerPoint and was not skilled in creating sophisticated image presentations). Nevertheless, by attending to the immediate presence of the images projected, it seemed as though the audience members were pressing me, in concert, to reconsider the complexity of what Immanuel Kant might have meant by the disinterested interest that one disposes toward an aesthetic object.

Upon returning to North America, the force of my audience's insistences gained greater political urgency when the Abu Ghraib photographs were published and circulated throughout the world. Though the outrage surrounding the scandal of torture (and the nihilistic cynicism of using torture as a means to defend democratic ideals) was not (and is not) at all irrelevant, such outrage is insufficient in explaining the effect of viewing those images. Or, to put the matter slightly differently, the images were striking regardless of the television caption or news headline that might have accompanied them.

The Abu Ghraib story broke when (on April 28, 2004) the CBS news program "60 Minutes 2" broadcast several of the photographs that showed U.S. GIs engaged in abusive acts and acts of dehumanization directed towards Iraqi prisoners. In the May 3, 2004 issue of *The New Yorker*, the photographs appeared in print for the first time and the subsequent week, *The New Yorker*'s Seymour Hersh published an article in the Annals of Security section of the magazine entitled "Torture at Abu Ghraib," where he detailed not only the acts of torture but the military investigation that followed.[1] *The New Yorker* had obtained a copy of what has since been referred to as the U.S. military's "Taguba Report,"[2] which, in its original variant, did not include the images in question because of their "extremely sensitive nature."[3] But the omission of the images in the Taguba Report is multifariously curious since, as Hersh rightly asserts, "the photographs tell it all."[4] The "all" that they tell, however, is not simply the story of military torture. Rather it's almost as if the report and the images stand in tension with one another, and that if the report had not appeared the images would have sufficed in their uncircumscribability. That is, "the photographs tell it all" neither because they are self-sufficient artifacts nor because they present the visible elements of what is seeable (i.e., the evidence of torture and humiliation) but because they present that which is not visible and yet palpable in an appearance.

As these are ongoing ruminations of mine, the possibility of closing off my discussion on a definitive note seems artificial. Thus I want to bring these reflections to a temporary repose by returning to some undeveloped comments that I make in my introductory remarks, in the hope of thinking further about the problems raised by the Abu Ghraib photographs. In those pages, and throughout this book, I introduce and deploy the term *organolepsis* to refer to the correspondences between perception and signification. More specifically, I also use the term to refer to the manner in which the external world impacts our lives and, through such experiences, compels a reconfiguration of our perceptual competencies. Given my initial assertion that politics is the activity of rendering perceptible those heterological elements that had previously been insensible, my concern has been to consider what are the organoleptic conditions of perceptibility for a political appearance.

In this respect, I affirmed that recognition is an inadequate ethical response to the emergence of a new political subjectivity because recognition implies an established context or field of reference that would act as a bannister of perceptual orientation. I also asserted that the experience of sensation that arises from the impact of an appearance is such that it disfigures or disarticulates those organoleptic assurances that would make recognition possible. Rather than recognition, then, I suggested that the emergence of a political appearance requires an act of admission: an appearance advenes upon us, and we admit to it. An act of recognition might follow from the durational intensity of advenience, but it does not follow causally in that there is no necessary condition that makes it so that I must (or even can) recognize any or all appearances.[5]

The appearance of the Abu Ghraib photographs is an event of advenience. I borrow the language of advenience from Roland Barthes's reflections on photography in his last work, *Camera Lucida*. In those pages Barthes introduces the now-famous distinction between a photograph's *studium* and its *punctum* in an attempt to at once distinguish and dismiss some of his previous work (especially the intertextual approach he masterfully lays out in *Image, Music, Text*). The distinction between the studium and the punctum lies in the difference between the general layout of a photograph (or the context of visibility that it offers) and its "point" which will "disturb" the studium. "A photograph's *punctum*," he asserts, "is that accident which pricks me (but also bruises me, is poignant to me)."[6] The rest of the short volume is dedicated to an exploration of what this distinction holds for Barthes, and how the experience of arrest plays itself out with other photographs. In other words, the point of that book is to engage the attraction people have to appearances that cannot be fully explained by justifying the frame of reference or the context of meaning. Barthes calls the force of attraction that sets off the disturbance of the punctum an *advenience*: "This picture *advenes*, that one doesn't."[7]

He doesn't say anything else about it other than to assert that the advenience of the image is also an adventure that animates him, but then he practically forgets about the term for the rest of the book. Nevertheless, it remains crucial to Barthes's reflections as it is the starting point for a set of considerations regarding an ethics of appearance.[8] How and why does one attend to an appearance? What is the intensity that does the work of capture, arrest, or conviction in an appearance such that it might compel us to have to recount the experience? Barthes's ruminations leave these questions open ended, and his commitment to the studium–punctum distinction, though insightful, does not satisfy the need to explain the complexity of advenience. But maybe that is precisely the point. That is, the force of an appearance and its presentation upon us does not require or expect a justification. An appearance advenes at me (not for me) and at best, my response can be one of admission. I admit to the appearance, to the monstrance of a new image or political subjectivity, not because I am obligated to recognize it and give it a name, but because it is present before me.[9]

I take this to be a first step in appreciating the intensity of the Abu Ghraib photographs that, for lack of a better expression, struck a chord.[10] The appearance of those photographs was much more significant than simply their status as evidentiary support for what everyone already knew: that physical torture and degradation is an all too common military policy.[11] Rather, the advenience of those photographs points to a fundamental ethical problem that concerns contemporary democratic life: namely, how to relate to an appearance and how to conceive an ethics of appearances when its presence disfigures or disarticulates our received normative inheritances; when an appearance, that is, punctures us.[12]

If, then, politics begins with the advenience of an appearance—with the rendering perceptible of a previously insensible—it is compelling to consider how we face up to appearances when their singularity affronts our particularities. We can refer to such felicitous affronts as instances of "cultural interface" that, as Lev Manovich explains, include the interaction with a computer keyboard or monitor, the viewing of a movie, or the cut-and-paste technology of word-processing software. Manovich's specific interest with such forms of cultural interface regards the development of "new sets of conventions for organizing data,"[13] and the repercussions of such conventions when thinking about how individuals relate to the world. But we can extend his account and consider cultural interface as an ethopoetic practice that involves ways of conceiving the relationship between individuals and appearances and takes the advenience of an appearance as an event of world making. Thus we can ask: what are the ethopoetic practices of cultural interface that constitute contemporary citizen subjects as subjects of perception?

This question has guided my explorations of the political life of sensation in these pages. As political life continues to be more and more complicit in acts of image-creation and transmission, it becomes increasingly urgent that we engage the strategies of perceptual competence that allow appearances to count as sensible. My ambition throughout this book has been to address this issue by shifting the focus of theoretical attention from a commitment to symbolic or interpretive signification to an analysis of the practices of perception in political life. For I take it to be of critical importance that before we may speak either of the meaning or qualitative value of any political claim, identity, or subjectivity, we habitually take as given certain perceptual assemblages that render a claim or subject available to our attentions. The observant and exhaustive concentration on what an appearance signifies, I have argued in my critique of narratocracy, overshadows the potential that lies in the act of appearing. Thus if we want to continue to conceive of political life as fundamentally tied to the emergence of an appearance—if individuals disposed toward a politically inflected mode of theoretical reflection continue to be equally disposed to the theatrocracy of democratic life—then we would be well served to consider the conditions of perceptual competence that act as limits to participation and as guarantors of an exclusivity that disable or delimit access to democratic forms of aesthetic and political part-taking. To say this is to suggest that the advenience of an appearance is a political event not because it is meaningful but because it acts upon our perceptual competencies and invites a turning of our attentions and a reconfiguration of those correspondences that mediate our worldly interactions. Such acts of attention and reconfiguration, I submit, are the ethical challenge of the political life of sensation.

NOTES

Prologue

Epigraph is from Maurice Merleau-Ponty, "Cézanne's Doubt," 15.

1 Here, and throughout this book, I engage Jacques Rancière's thesis that "politics is aesthetic in that it makes visible what had been excluded from a perceptual field, and that it makes audible what had been inaudible." Rancière, *The Philosopher and His Poor*, 226.

2 I will have more to say about the tasting subject and its role in the history of political thought in chapter 5.

3 Organoleptic: (from *organ* + Greek *lēptikos* meaning disposed to take or accept, to seize). "Of, relating to, or involving the use of sense organs or senses, especially of smell and taste." *Oxford English Dictionary Online*, s.v. "organoleptic." The *lēptikos* of organolepsis, I should specify, also refers to how the external world impacts our sensory organs, how these same sensory organs are formed by the impact of percepts, and to the correspondences between a sense organ and acts of perception: we know that our eyes grant us sight, and it would be unimaginable to conceive of visuality as a form of touching. And yet, as I elaborate in chapter 4, Aloïs Riegl's studies on the aesthetic and historical value of ancient monuments and sculptures determined the importance of haptic visuality, of the eye's caress, when approaching such artifacts. In the case of Riegl and many other political theorists, cultural activists, and artists discussed in these pages, the heterogeneity of perception suggests a disarticulation of the correspondences that bind a sense organ to an act of perception.

This theme of the heterogeneity of perception (especially as regards vision and touch) is also taken up by Jean-Luc Nancy when, at the end of his *Noli me tangere: Essai sur la levée du corps*, he poses the following set of questions: "But what is vision if not anything less than a deferred touch? And what is a deferred touch if not a touch that intensifies or distills without repose, to the point of a necessary excess, the point, the prick of a point, and the moment when the touch distances itself from what has been touched, at the very moment when touching occurs?" (81–82) The original French reads as follows: "Mais qu'est ce que la vue, sinon, sans doute, un toucher différé? Mais qu'est-ce qu'un toucher différé, sinon un toucher qui aiguise ou qui distille sans réserve, jusqu'à un excès nécessaire, le point, la pointe et l'instant par quoi la touche se détache de ce qu'elle touche, au moment même où elle le touche?" My translation.

4 Foucault, *The Hermeneutics of the Subject*, 243. In the second part of the Collège de France seminar of February 10, 1982, Foucault expands on what he means by *ethopoesis* by distinguishing between pointless and useful knowledge. Discussing the writings of Demetrius, he explains that pointless knowledge is the kind of knowledge that pursues hidden causes, like the hidden causes that permit the birth of twins, or those involved in optical illusions. These are pointless, however, not because an acquisition of such knowledge ought to be prohibited but because "they are to be known, if we wish to know them, only as an extra, as it were, when the soul *in tutum retracto* (withdrawn into that region of security which provides it with wisdom), wants additionally to seek out these causes, as diversion and in order to find a pleasure precisely solely in discovery itself" (234). The things useful to know, and the forms of knowledge that Foucault wants to pursue, are the ones that relate to the world as a common dwelling place. Knowledge is in this way useful when it is oriented towards ethos-formation. Thus we have ethopoesis: "a relational mode of knowledge that asserts and prescribes at the same time and is capable of producing a change in the subject's mode of being" (238).

Relevant to this discussion is the fact that the discourse of ethopoesis lies between what Foucault calls the Platonic *epistrophē* (or turning away from appearances) and the Christian *metanoia* (the conversion, whose fundamental element is a renunciation of oneself for the sake of a rebirth). The distinction that ethopoesis offers is that it is neither a turning away from appearances (*epistrophē*) nor a rejection of a former self (*metanoia*). On the contrary, ethopoesis refers to a mode of interface with the world of appearances that produces a transformation in our subjectivities which is at once a dissolution and rearticulation of ourselves. As a relational mode of knowledge, it is fundamentally invested in that which makes interactivity possible, and it is a mode of knowing that takes bodily practices of living as sources for the kinds of connections, affinities, and resonances we at once engage and refuse.

Foucault's emphasis in these pages is on ethos-formation, a point that many scholars have noted marks a substantive shift in his thinking and research from the kinds of motivations that structured his investigations on disciplinarity and governmentality. Most recently, Judith Butler has contrasted Foucault's discussion of morality in this later period from that of Nietzsche. Rather than a limit to one's self-crafting (as in the case of Nietzsche) for Foucault "what relation the self will take to itself, how it will craft itself in response to an injunction, how it will form itself and what labor it will perform on itself is a challenge, if not an open question" (Butler, *Giving an Account of Oneself*, 18). The open-endedness that Butler finds in Foucault rests on a point of fundamental importance: namely, that there is never a moment that we are free from those kinds of conditions (call them norms or injunctions) that might arrest us. What becomes ethically significant, therefore, is not the nature of the injunction per se but our turnings and re-turnings around those instances of arrest, those moments of interruption in our daily lives, that compel us to reconfigure our perceptual and organoleptic arrangements.

5 Here I allude to what Hannah Arendt called a "thinking without a bannister" (*Hannah Arendt*, 336). For Arendt, the faculty of judgment intervened when bannisters were not available. I am suggesting that more than thinking without a bannister, individuals are often faced with the task of judging without bannisters, without, that is, standards or rules for judgment.

6 For my interests, the studies done by Kaja Silverman in *The Threshold of the Visible World* and Slavoj Žižek in *Looking Awry* and *The Sublime Object of Ideology* are of particular importance. Nevertheless, my orientation in this book shares greater affinities with the kinds of concerns that William Connolly (in *Neuropolitics*), Gregory Flaxman (in his edited volume, *The Brain is the Screen*), Laura Marks (in *The Skin of the Film*), Michael Shapiro (in *Deforming American Political Thought*), Steven Shaviro (in *The Cinematic Body*), and Vivian Sobchak (in *Carnal Thoughts*) raise in their analyses of the relationship between the body, perception, aesthetics, and politics.

7 Massumi, *Parables for the Virtual*, 3.

8 Arendt, *Eichmann in Jerusalem*, 262.

9 See for instance the diverse and rich body of research included in Jodi Dean's edited volume *Cultural Studies and Political Theory*.

10 A variety of thinkers come to mind in this respect—most notably Judith Butler, Julia Kristeva, and Luce Irigaray. However, for the purposes of these introductory reflections, I am particularly indebted to Iris Marion Young's essay, "Throwing Like a Girl: A Phenomenology of Feminine Body Comportment, Motility, and Spatiality," and her appropriation of Merleau-Ponty's notion of the lived body to discuss feminine forms of bodily existence. In that essay Young is especially persuasive in her treatment of the place of visuality—what she refers to as the "threat of being seen" (45)—when discussing the relationship between action, mobility, and perception. I distance myself from Young's discussion at precisely the point where she expresses anxiety about the element of discontinuity in feminine bodily existence.

11 At the outset, I want to make clear that this project is not a critique of visuality per se but is, rather, an appreciation of the fact that the implicit commitment to vision in much contemporary political thought is accompanied by an inattentiveness to the theories of visuality that such a commitment endorses.

12 Taylor, "The Politics of Recognition" in *Multiculturalism*, 64.

13 Patchen Markell's *Bound by Recognition* provides an excellent engagement with the sovereigntist dimensions of a politics of recognition and the "posture of confident mastery" (12) that accompanies the pursuit of an ideal of recognition. My interest here is less in the subjugating power dynamics involved in the conceptual analysis of the politics of recognition than in the account of visuality that is at once absent and necessary for the dialectics of recognition to function.

14 On various treatments of figuration in contemporary aesthetics, see D. N. Rodowick's *Reading the Figural, or, Philosophy after the New Media*.

15 See Taylor's "Interpretation and the Sciences of Man."

16 I discuss these and other aspects of Rancière's thought throughout and in chapter 1 extensively. For a concise and insightful treatment of Rancière on aesthetic regimes of perception, see Rockhill, "The Silent Revolution."

17 Rancière, *The Politics of Aesthetics*, 12.

18 Panagia and Rancière, "Dissenting Words," 115.

19 Erin Manning, *The Politics of Touch*, 13.

20 Gilles Deleuze's work on Francis Bacon is especially relevant to this discussion and specifically his treatment of Antonin Artaud's "body without organs" thesis: "A wave with variable amplitude flows through the body without organs," he explains, "it traces zones and levels on this body according to the variations of its amplitude. When the wave encounters external forces at a particular level, a sensation appears. An organ will be determined by this encounter, but it is a provisional organ that endures only as long as the passage of the wave and the action of the force, and which will be displaced in order to be posited elsewhere." Gilles Deleuze, *Francis Bacon*, 41.

21 Morrone, Ross, and Burr, "Saccadic eye movements cause compression of time as well as space," 951.

22 Ibid., 952.

23 I would like to specify before I proceed that my discussion of Merleau-Ponty's account of Cézanne should not suggest that Merleau-Ponty provides the definitive account of Cézanne's oeuvre. There are many other accounts worth considering. However, and for the purposes of these considerations, my interest is in Merleau-Ponty's distinction between an outline and a contour that he finds in the works of Cézanne, which I think is also relevant to political reflection. For an extended treatment of Merleau-Ponty's political thought, see Diana Coole's *Merleau-Ponty and Modern Politics after Anti-Humanism*, especially her discussion of "the generativity of the flesh" (164–81).

24 Maurice Merleau-Ponty, "Cézanne's Doubt," 11.

25 Ibid., 13.

26 The geometrical perspective finds its classic analysis in Erwin Panofsky's *Perspective as Symbolic Form* which describes this "central perspective" ("central" in the sense of visually attending to the center of the image, as in the case of the vanishing point) as having two essential but tacit assumptions: "first, that we see with a single and immobile eye, and second, that the planar cross section of the visual pyramid can pass as an adequate reproduction of our optical image" (29).

27 Merleau-Ponty, "Cézanne's Doubt," 14–15.

28 Ibid., 15.

29 Deleuze, *Francis Bacon*, especially chapter 6, "Painting and Sensation" (31–38).

30 Merleau-Ponty, *Phenomenology of Perception*, 10.

31 Ibid., 62.

32 Giovanni Garroni, *Elogio dell'imprecisione*, 7. The Italian reads as follows: "Ciò che c'è di indeterminato negli oggetti costituisce quel bordo ambiguo che permette le sovrapposizioni, le allusioni e anche le confusioni. Questa instabilità sottrae gli oggetti alla solitudine, cui li condannerebbe una ipotetica precisione assoluta." My translation.

33 I take the tension between these two poles of Arendt's thought—between appearance and representation—to be compelling and frustrating at the same time given the ease with which she relies on narrative emplotment as a solution for rendering action at once visible and permanent. See Arendt's treatment of storytelling in *The Human Condition* (especially pages 184–88). Also see Paul Ricoeur's discussion of emplotment and threefold mimesis in *Time and Narrative*.

34 de Certeau, *The Writing of History*, 89.

35 The phrase "organization of the visible" is borrowed from Jonathan Crary's study on technologies of visuality in the nineteenth century, *Techniques of the Observer*, 23.

36 Butler, "Endangered / Endangering," 205.

37 Ibid., 205.

38 Ibid.

39 Ibid., 210.

40 I will expand on Vivian Sobchack's felicitous phrase, "the viewing subject" in chapter 4. For Sobchack's treatment of it, see her work *The Address of the Eye*, especially 97–127.

41 In her recent discussion of Adriana Cavarero's work, Judith Butler has forwarded a critique of the role of narrative in ethical accountability. See Butler, *Giving an Account of Oneself*, especially 30–40.

42 The emphasis on filmic techniques of production is what I take to be the lesson of Michael Moore's *Fahrenheit 9/11*. In this respect, the most disappointing thing about the reactions to that movie was the incessant focus on the film's content. It seemed that there were only two possible responses to it: spectators either chose to side with Moore's heavy-handed Bush attacks or criticize him for being even more conspiratorial than Oliver Stone. Either way, the story line was the focus of appraisal. But in doing so, media critics, political pundits, and moviegoers alike endorsed precisely the point that Moore was trying to condemn. That is, *Fahrenheit 9/11* is not a movie that tells a story; it is a movie about the telling of stories. In other words, it is a movie that points to the power of editing as an image-making technique.

This is most evident in Moore's almost annoying (though humorous) treatment of George W. Bush in the first half of the movie. The cajoling and derision of the president is so over the top—even for Moore's standards—that one cannot help but wonder if he is not trying to do something else with it. It's almost as if Moore wants us to see how easy it is to tell half-truths. Consider, for instance, the clip that introduces the Bush administration using the "Bonanza" opening credit sequence, or the scene that shows Bush committed to reading a children's story after having been informed of the 9 / 11 attacks. No one can actually take such images too seriously and, given their tone, you are not meant to. There is something else at work and at stake here for Moore.

That something else is the condition of the modern citizen subject qua viewing subject (see chapter 4). *Fahrenheit 9/11* is edited, cut, and pasted in such a transparent manner that it makes the processes of editing, cutting, and pasting themselves the central characters of the movie, not only the Bush presidency. Moreover, it makes all those dismissive criticisms of the movie as heavy handed and conspiratorial entirely off the mark; or rather, these criticisms are, themselves, part of the failure of contemporary media literacy. The kind of blind faith that emphasizes information over exposition, content over form, literally blinds us to the narratocratic technologies of presentation, of which editing is the most dramatic. As a result, we tend to fall into the pattern of simply taking sides without ever questioning what compels us to make those judgments something like what happened to the Simi Valley jurors in the Rodney King trial.

43 Wittgenstein, *Philosophical Investigations*, paragraph 161.

44 On the aesthetic dimensions of Wittgenstein's duck-rabbit example and its relation to political judgment, see Kennan Ferguson's discussion in his *The Politics of Judgment*, especially 17–23 and 85–91.

45 Linda Zerilli, *Feminism and the Abyss of Freedom*, 55.

46 Ibid., 56.

47 For a helpful treatment of the connections and differences between my work and Linda Zerilli's, see Tarnopolsky, "Platonic Reflections on the Aesthetic Dimensions of Deliberative Democracy."

48 Zerilli, *Feminism and the Abyss of Freedom*, 59. On a related point, or set of points, on the role of the imagination in political thinking, see Drucilla Cornell's discussion of what she calls "conjectural participation" in *Defending Ideals*, especially 41–62.

49 In a recent essay critical of Pierre Bourdieu's sociology of aesthetics, Jacques Rancière has been explicit about this debt to Kant. See Rancière's "Thinking between Disciplines."

50 I take this point to be an extension of Hayden White's seminal

analysis of emplotment in *Metahistory*. Also see White's forward to Rancière's *The Names of History*.

Chapter One

Epigraph from Kant, *Critique of Judgment*, trans. J. H. Bernard, first part, section 34.

1 Deleuze, "To Have Done with Judgment."

2 Ibid., 135.

3 Indistinction is an important historical problem in the philosophy of art which looks to the role of forgeries and the forms of knowledge required in order to distinguish a fake from the original. Recent developments in twentieth-century art have complicated the question of indistinction to the extent that artists like Andy Warhol, Marcel Duchamp, and Jasper Johns established conditions of indistinguishability between art and ordinary objects, compelling us to ask that "if in theory *everything* can be art, then how is it possible to distinguish between art and non-art?" Sándor Radnóti, *The Fake*, 126; see also Arthur Danto's *The Transfiguration of the Commonplace*. Though Deleuze is not explicit about his debt to this tradition of reflection, these debates are nonetheless important for understanding the implication of Deleuze's own elaborations on indistinction, especially given his philosophical and aesthetic commitment to the problematic of the simulacra vis-à-vis the doctrine of judgment.

4 Deleuze, "Bartleby; or, The Formula," 71.

5 For an insightful philosophical engagement with this impasse, see Katharine Wolfe's treatment in "From Aesthetics to Politics."

6 Rancière, "Deleuze, Bartleby, and the Literary Formula," 161. The passage from Deleuze's essay to which Rancière refers is the following: "A contemporary of American transcendentalism (Emerson, Thoreau), Melville is already sketching out the traits of the pragmatism that will be its continuation. It is first of all the affirmation of a world in *process*, an *archipelago*. Not even a puzzle, whose pieces when fitted together would constitute a whole, but rather a wall of loose, uncemented stones, where every element has a value in itself but also in relation to others: isolated and floating relations, islands and straits, immobile points and sinuous lines—for Truth has always had 'jagged edges'." Deleuze, "Bartleby; or, The Formula," 86.

7 Ibid., 162.

8 Part of my interest is to rethink the role of Kantian aesthetic judgment in political reflection and the manner in which it is too often associated with the sharing of communal values as the basis for the pronouncement of judgments. Though I depart from his account, I am grateful for Kennan Ferguson's explorations of similar themes in his *The Politics of Judgment*. I am also indebted to him for comments he provided on an earlier version of this chapter.

9 See Paul Guyer's discussion of disinterest in the eighteenth century in his *Kant and the Experience of Freedom*.

10 Steven Shaviro makes some similar remarks regarding Kant in his essay "Beauty Lies in the Eye."

11 Huntington, "The Clash of Civilizations?"

12 Hutcheson, *An Inquiry into the Original of Our Ideas of Beauty and Virtue*, 19.

13 Guyer, *Kant and the Experience of Freedom*, 59.

14 As I argue below, Kant's own account of "disinterested interest" is not synonymous with Shaftesbury's aristocratic ideal of aesthetic detachment but a critique of it.

15 Kant, *Critique of Judgment*, first part, section 5. From this point on the citations are from the Oxford translation. The material in the square brackets is my addition to the quotation, and it refers to the designations Kant makes a few lines earlier in this same section.

16 As Jonathan Crary has shown, claims about spectatorship, observation, and impartiality are characteristic of middle to late nineteenth-century techniques of visuality that, I am implying, would not have been available to Immanuel Kant. Indeed, Kant's writings may be comfortably situated within the regime of visuality that Crary associates with the camera obscura and not with that of the stereoscope. Thus, "the achievement of that kind of optical neutrality, the reduction of the observer to a supposedly rudimentary state, was both an aim of artistic experimentation of the second half of the nineteenth century *and* a condition for the formation of the observer who would be competent to consume vast new amounts of visual imagery and information increasingly circulated during this same period. It was the remaking of the visual field not into a tabula rasa on which orderly representations could be arrayed, but into a surface of inscription on which a promiscuous range of effects could be produced. The visual culture of modernity would coincide with such techniques of the observer." Crary, *Techniques of the Observer*, 96.

17 Kant, *Critique of Judgment*, first part, section 4.

18 See Frances Ferguson's discussion of utilitarian representational structures in her *Pornography, the Theory*, especially 3–5.

19 Kant, *Critique of Judgment*, first part, section 5.

20 "We must not be in the least prejudiced," Kant asserts, "in favor of the existence of the things, but be quite indifferent in this respect, in order to play the judge in things of taste." Ibid., first part, section 2.

21 Ibid., first part, section 12; "linger" is the term used in the Cambridge University Press translation of the *Critique of Judgment*.

22 By this, I take Kant to be accounting for the kind of common experience many of us might have had when being told by a reliable source that a movie is excellent and must be seen. Once we do see that movie, we remain somewhat disappointed because it did not live up to our expectations.

23 Ibid., first part, section 4.

24 Ibid., first part, section 8. My emphasis.

25 I use Wittgenstein's language from the *Philosophical Investigations* to discuss Kant's claim because there is, I think, a profound sympathy between these two thinkers on this matter. Indeed, the not implausible claim could be made that in Wittgenstein's discussion of rule and rule following one finds an indebtedness to Kant's antinormative stance vis-à-vis aesthetic judgment. Or, at the very least, one could say that they are talking about the same experience.

26 It might seem to some that the problem with my account of Kantian aesthetic experience is that I am collapsing the distinction between an experience of the beautiful and of the sublime. In a sense I am doing just that, to the extent that at the moment of aesthetic experience I think that Kant believes that the distinction is unavailable to us. It is only after the fact, once we determine either pleasure or pain, that we are able to categorize the experience as one of the beautiful or of the sublime. In other words, the only real difference between these two moments comes in the form of the character of the sensation (either pleasant or painful) but not in the conditions of aesthetic experience.

27 For more on Deleuze's debt to Kant, see Smith, "Deleuze, Kant, and the Theory of Immanent Ideas."

28 In the chapter entitled "The Banality of the Negative" of my *The Poetics of Political Thinking*, I conclude with the problem of judgment in Deleuze's thought but leave the matter suspended. Here, I want to pick up on where that discussion leaves off.

29 Deleuze, "To Have Done with Judgment," 126.

30 Deleuze links the doctrine of judgment with the Judeo-Christian theological tradition of having a debt to God. Ibid., 126–27.

31 Ibid., 129.

32 This ontological position is admirably treated by Smith in his essay, "Deleuze's Theory of Sensation." Attending to Deleuze's notion of intensity, Smith describes what I am calling Deleuze's ontology of sensation thusly: "beyond prepared matter lies an energetic materiality in continuous variation, and beyond fixed form lie qualitative processes of deformation and transformation in continuous development" (43).

33 Rancière, "Deleuze, Bartleby, and the Literary Formula," 157.

34 At this point, and as an aside, I wish to foreground the fact that my reading of Deleuze throughout these pages is informed by his work on David Hume in his *Empiricism and Subjectivity* as well as *Difference and Repetition*. It is Deleuze's Humeanism that marks his commitment to empiricism as the source for an appreciation of affect. There is a strong connection between Deleuze's thought and eighteenth-century accounts of sensation, and this connection is the basis of my understanding of Deleuze's ontology of sensation.

35 In this regard he states: "At bottom, a doctrine of judgment presumes that the gods give *lots* to men and that men, depending on their lots, are fit for some particular form. For some particular organic end." Deleuze, "To Have Done with Judgment," 129.

36 Deleuze, *Difference and Repetition*, 33.

37 Kant, *Critique of Judgment*, first part, section 40. In *The Poetics of Political Thinking* I also discuss Kant's *sensus communis* in the context of what I call a "Rawlsian Aesthetic" and with regards to the elements of comparison and accountability in John Rawls's image of political thought. Because my interest in that discussion is to elaborate on the tacit aesthetic conditions of contemporary political argument, I completely omit the durational dimensions of aesthetic judgment that interest me here.

38 Ibid., second part, section 59.

39 Deleuze, *Kant's Critical Philosophy*, 68.

40 Paul Guyer's more favorable account of this point is the following: "it is precisely in virtue of the freedom of the imagination in aesthetic response from determination by ordinary concepts of the understanding that this response is itself suited to serve as a symbol of morality, because it can thereby represent the freedom that is the essence of morality, yet which is not otherwise made palpable to us in the world of our senses." *Values of Beauty*, 7.

41 Deleuze, *Difference and Repetition*, 33.

42 Deleuze, "To Have Done with Judgment," 129.

43 Deleuze and Guattari, *A Thousand Plateaus*, 497.

44 I am here referring to, among other things, the idea of "sentence meaning" developed by Jeremy Bentham in his *Theory of Fictions* and subsequently picked up by Wittgenstein, Austin, and Derrida in their relative attempts to account for the relationship of words and sentences. For an engagement with Bentham on this issue, see Frances Ferguson's discussion in *Pornography*, 3.

45 Saint-Exupéry, *Le Petit Prince*.

46 Smith, "Deleuze's Theory of Sensation," 41.

47 Deleuze and Guattari, *A Thousand Plateaus*, 497–98 (emphasis in original).

48 This is the basis of Deleuze's discussion of figuration in his *Francis Bacon* that I take up in chapter 4.

49 Deleuze, *Difference and Repetition*, 303.

50 Rancière, *The Politics of Aesthetics*, 15.

51 Rancière, *The Philosopher and His Poor*, 225.

52 I discuss this further in chapter 4. Rancière's distinction between the police and politics is discussed throughout his writings but especially in *Dis-Agreement*, "Ten Theses on Politics," and Panagia and Rancière, "Dissenting Words." I present an account of the aesthetic features of these concepts in my *The Poetics of Political Thinking*.

53 Deleuze and Guattari, *A Thousand Plateaus*, 158.

54 Rancière, *The Philosopher and His Poor*, 226.

55 Ibid.

56 Deleuze, *Difference and Repetition*, 34.

57 Rancière, "Deleuze, Bartleby, and the Literary Formula," 162.

Chapter Two

The first epigraph is from Erasmus, *Praise of Folly*, 7. The second epigraph is from de Certeau, "Vocal Utopias," 30.

1 Sarno, "EU Chocolate Vote Threatens Cocoa Producers."

2 Rancière, *The Philosopher and His Poor*, 47.

3 Saussure, *Course in General Linguistics*, 66.

4 McLuhan, *Understanding Media*, 32. McLuhan's observations regarding the literary bias of our culture still ring true today as John

Guillory's recent "The Memo and Modernity" clearly shows. In this essay, Guillory provides a fascinating account of "the generic features of informational writing by focusing on a single genre—the memorandum—the humblest yet perhaps the most ubiquitous genre of writing in the modern world," 111.

5 Imagine how utterly senseless it must have sounded to French aristocrats to hear common people referring to themselves as "*citoyens*"—a new word inserted within a political reality that was still to come. Or, for that matter, how entirely Babelian St. Paul's letters that spoke of a redeeming Christ, human divinity, and the sacred body of the Church must have sounded to the ears of the Corinthians.

6 Michael Warner, *Publics and Counterpublics*, 114.

7 Barthes, "The Grain of the Voice." The grain of the voice for Barthes refers to the "very precise space of the encounter between a language and a voice" (181).

8 Chartier, *The Order of Books*, 8.

9 Ginzburg, *The Cheese and the Worms*.

10 Chartier, *The Order of Books*, 12.

11 Rawls, *Political Liberalism*, xxiv.

12 Rancière, *The Names of History*, 89.

13 de Certeau, *The Writing of History*, 47.

14 Ibid., 73.

15 Ginzburg, *The Cheese and the Worms*, xxvi.

16 Struever, *Theory as Practice*, 168.

17 See Olga Zorzi Pugliese's discussion of dialogism in Castiglione in Pugliese, "L'evoluzione della struttura dialogica nel *Libro del cortegiano*," 59–68.

18 Struever, *Theory as Practice*, 175.

19 Arendt, *The Human Condition*, 15

20 Rancière, *Dis-Agreement*, 50.

21 See Bataille, "The Notion of Expenditure," as well as his more extensive treatment of the idea of nonproductive expenditure in *The Accursed Share*. For a more sustained anthropology of *potlatch*, see Marcel Mauss's *The Gift*.

22 Skinner, "Meaning and Understanding in the History of Ideas," 82. Hereafter, all citations from Skinner will be from his *Visions of Politics*, citing the page number but not the specific essay whence they are extracted.

23 Skinner, *Visions of Politics*, 2.

24 Ibid., 115.

25 Ibid.

26 See "The Practice of History and the Cult of the Fact" in ibid., passim.

27 Skinner, *Visions of Politics*, 54.

28 Ibid., 42.

29 Ibid., 82.

30 Ibid., 54.

31 Ibid., 55.

32 Ibid.

33 de Certeau, *The Writing of History*, 72.

34 Ibid., 3.

35 Ibid., 2.

36 This, in turn, ties into a tradition of rhetoric that distinguishes between the serious and authoritative voice of knowledge and the mad and frivolous babble of folly, as the Erasmus epigraph suggests.

37 Kandinsky, *Point and Line to Plane*, 101.

38 Kandinsky, *Concerning the Spiritual in Art*, passim but especially the chapter on colors.

39 Kandinsky, *Point and Line to Plane*, 57. What seems relevant to me about Kandinsky's paintings is that by emphasizing the distinction between point and line, they also emphasize the artistic dimension of the grapheme so that within the context of a discussion of the somatic dimensions of reading and writing, Kandinsky provides purchase on the importance of something like the choice of fonts one chooses when writing using word-processing software. For someone like Kandinsky, it would matter to one's argument as a whole whether one chose Times Roman font over Courier New font because both of these modes of graphic representation suggest different experiences of duration in the manner in which each font follows and shapes a line differently. An historical corollary to this is the role of illuminators in the preparation of manuscripts in the early-modern period. For a particularly engaging case study of medieval illustrators, see Michael Camille's *Image on the Edge*. Not to be overlooked in this regard is Michael Fried's discussion in his book *Realism, Writing, Disfiguration* of the contrast between writing or drawing and painting in Thomas Eakins's *The Gross Clinic*. Whereas Fried convincingly shows how Eakins's painting establishes a sharp division between the horizontal topography of writing or drawing and that of painting (the vertical plane of the canvas), I want to suggest that by

shifting our attention to the durational aspects of the line, Kandinsky wants to suture the division drawn by the realist tradition.

40 Saussure, *Course in General Linguistics*, 66.

41 Ibid..

42 Ibid., 70.

43 With this I want to suggest that Skinner's slippage into a history of "true beliefs" is, in large part, a result of treating historical texts as static objects. Though I concur with Skinner's claim regarding the performative character of speech acts and the importance of context in historical analysis, his observations are circumscribed by his limiting the utterances' potential to that of the signified or, indeed, in making the utterance exclusively an instance of *disputatio*.

44 Bakhtin, "The Problem of Speech Genres," 63.

45 Ibid., 69.

46 Ibid., 71.

47 Ibid., 72.

48 Ibid., 79.

49 Arendt, *Responsibility and Judgment*, 12.

50 My understanding of democratic nonsense finds affinity with Brent Hayes Edwards's discussion of "scat semantics" in "Louis Armstrong and the Syntax of Scat." Most notably, I am taken with the way Edwards connects the origins of scat with the apocryphal "dropping of words" story retold by Louis Armstrong along with the latter's obsession with scatological release.

51 In *The Shape of the Signifier*, Walter Benn Michaels notes how glossolalia is a recurrent theme in much 1990s American science fiction writing and concludes that it is a way of talking about a language "while bypassing meaning" (83). His treatment of this phenomenon is noteworthy because of his attack on the materialist view of language and textuality and his claim that such materialisms are interested in experiences of texts and not interpretations of them. Thus, Michaels conflates a de Manian "materialist vision" of the text with a pluralist account of meaning, concluding that the difference between experience and interpretation is the difference between identity and belief, which is the difference between "difference-as-such" and disagreement. In the end, poststructural accounts of politics make disagreement impossible according to Michaels. (I discuss these issues further in my review of Michaels's book, "*The Shape of the Signifier* or, The Ontology of Argument.") Though there is much to admire and disagree with in Michaels's

compelling work, I want to specify that I am not arguing in favor of "meaningless speech," nor, do I think, is de Certeau in his treatment of glossolalia. Rather, what I want to suggest is that from the ideological position of an authoritative discursive regime, other modes of speaking will sound like babble or noise. Thus, the possibility of democratic non-sense as a speech genre of political interlocution does not refer to meaninglessness per se but to who gets to decide what meaninglessness sounds like.

52 See Rancière's thesis 5 in "Ten Theses on Politics."

53 de Certeau, "Vocal Utopias," 40.

54 Ibid., 30.

55 Ibid., 34.

56 Ibid., 39.

57 The Bible, Genesis 11:4.

58 *Oxford English Dictionary Online*, s.v. babel.

59 Here, I follow Rancière's analysis of democracy from thesis 5 of his "Ten Theses on Politics," where he states that "the people (*demos*) exists only as a rupture of the logic of *arche*, a rupture of the logic of beginning / ruling [*commencement / commandement*]. . . . The 'people' is the (abstract) supplement that inscribes 'the count of the unaccounted-for' or 'the part of those who have no part'."

60 Importantly, within the Christian tradition, the undoing of this curse is remembered on Pentecostal Sunday—the feast which recalls a day, after Christ's ascension, when the apostles were given the gift of the holy spirit and learned to speak in tongues—a glossolalia that allowed them to be heard preaching in whatever native language the listener enjoyed: "They were all filled with the Holy Spirit and began to talk in other languages, as the Spirit enabled them to speak." Acts of the Apostles, 2:1–5.

61 de Certeau, "Vocal Utopias," 30.

62 Sanga, "Campane e campanili," 38.

63 de Certeau, *The Practice of Everyday Life*, 117. "A space," de Certeau states, "exists when one takes into consideration vectors of direction, velocities, and time variables. . . . On this view, in relation to place, space is like a word when it is spoken, that is, when it is caught in the ambiguity of an actualization."

64 Ibid.

65 Romano, "Le piazze e i cittadini."

66 Isnenghi, *L'Italia in piazza*, 3. All translations of this and other Italian texts are my own.

67 Ibid., 5.

68 Sanga, "Campane e campanili," 48.

69 One of the best illustrations of this tension is found in the 1951 Italian film *Don Camillo*. Based on Giovanni Guareschi's novel *Il piccolo mondo di Don Camillo*, the movie recounts the story of the clash between the recently elected Communist mayor of Brescello (in the Po River Valley of northern Italy), Peppone (played by Gino Cervi), and the town's parish priest, Don Camillo (played by the French actor, Fernandel). The scene opens with the narrator's voice-over (in the dubbed English version, Orson Welles is the narrator) setting the stage: the "*piccolo mondo*" (small world) is a microcosm of the struggles that emerge in Italian politics after the formation of the Republic (1946).

A crane shot lands on the central town piazza. The scene is the acceptance speech of the recently elected Peppone who will introduce his "comrade" from the big city and who, in his turn, proceeds to orate on the struggle of the workers against the established autocracy of church and capital. Don Camillo, pacing furiously inside the church and already scandalized by the fact that the band playing the "Internazionale" is composed of those same students to whom he had taught music, expresses his outrage to the church's crucifix (with which he has a vivid dialogue throughout the movie). Suddenly, upon being reprimanded by the talking Jesus and told that what happens "out there" (in the piazza) is not his domain, Don Camillo disappears behind a large wooden door and is next seen atop the duomo's bell tower (still his domain), feverishly ringing the bells under the hot summer sun. The shot pans between the electronic microphone speakers on the orator's stage and the swinging of the bells, all the while showing the swaying of the spectators' heads between the two aural poles. Though comic, the poignancy of this scene lies in the anachronistic nexus established between the noise of the amplified microphone (a new medium) and that of the bell (the more ancient call). The locus of that nexus, where the two noises collide, is the piazza itself. Barely bearing this cacophony, the crowd is understandably bewildered not only because both sounds are incomprehensible (the orator's speech is completely overshadowed by the bells and the bells are being played out of time, out of synch, and out of tune) but also because, in that piazza, they stand at the disjuncture (both historical and geographic) of the separation of church and state and the birth of Italian secularism.

70 Sanga, "Campane e campanili," 40.

71 Ibid.

72 Isnenghi, *L'Italia in piazza*, 18.

73 Dondi, "Piazzale Loreto," 493.

74 Bakhtin, *Rabelais and His World*.

75 Dondi, "Piazzale Loreto," 495.

76 The edicola has a longer history than its modern status as a newsstand. Originally, edicolas were small carvings on buildings or street corners where the faithful would install relics of saints or religious icons, which would then stand as markers of devotional prayer. These earlier edicolas exist to this day in Italy. As a further note, there is a long history of the relationship between piazzas and print culture not only with regards to the religious history of Catholic art but also, and most recently, with regards to the development and proliferation of the political poster, which, as Luciano Celes notes, "is related to the outdoor nature of much recreational life in Italy: the ritual of the *passeggiata* (the walk) alone justifies the parties' investment in this form of communication." Celes, "Picture Battles in the Piazza," 125. In this discussion of the semiotics of modern political advertising in Italy, Celes also points out how the political poster attracts graffiti which invokes the Pasquinade tradition in Renaissance Rome, "the practice of writing comments and gossip on placards hanging from a statue located in a city-centre piazza" (125).

77 The story of the funding for this restoration project recounted in interviews I conducted with Orlandi (in February of 2004) is too long to discuss in this context. However, there is ample editorial documentation in the local papers as it was a topic of attention throughout the restoration process.

78 Bazzani, "Un mini-museo d'arte."

79 Bassi, "Chioschi: Appunti di storia e di quotidianità," 29.

80 Orlandi, "L'Arredo Urbano." Catalog published on the occasion of the "Età Progettuale" exhibit at the Istituto Santa Chiara, Casalmaggiore, March 18–May 14, 2006.

81 Interview with Marco Orlandi conducted by Davide Panagia, February 22, 2004.

82 Orlandi, *Edicola nel tempo*, 2.

83 Bolsi, "Acanto," 12. My translation.

84 de Certeau, *The Practice of Everyday Life*, 97.

85 Orlandi, *Edicola nel tempo*, 2. My translation.

86 Chartier, *The Order of Books*, 8.

87 de Certeau, "Vocal Utopias," 41.

Chapter Three

Epigraph is quoted in Camille, "Before the Gaze," 201.

1 Camille, "Before the Gaze," 197.

2 "Edicola" is derived from the Latin *aedicula*, a diminutive of *aedes* meaning "temple."

3 Strocchia, *Death and Ritual in Renaissance Florence*, 150.

4 In this respect, I agree with Konrad Eisenbichler's conclusion in his introduction to *Carnival and the Carnivalesque* that the study of carnival life is far from monolithic and that the variety of practices and activities in carnival life requires "a multiplicity of understandings, approaches, and interests" (16).

5 McCormick, "MACHIAVELLI AGAINST REPUBLICANISM," 637.

6 See Skinner's volume, *Visions of Politics*.

7 Skinner, "Interpretation and the Understanding of Speech Acts," 115. In this regard, he also states that "one of the most salutary achievements of post-modern cultural criticism has been to improve our awareness of the purely rhetorical aspects of writing and speech thereby heightening our sensitivity to the relations between language and power." *Visions of Politics*, 5.

8 Skinner, "Interpretation and the Understanding of Speech Acts," 115.

9 Viroli, "Machiavelli and the Republican Idea of Politics," 144.

10 Ibid.

11 Ibid., 145.

12 Ibid., 147.

13 Ibid., 152.

14 Ibid., 156.

15 Ibid., 160.

16 Ibid., 161.

17 Ibid., 163. The reason for this conclusion is that the vocabulary of "*stato*" is one of status, not of "the state," and this language is one that stands in contrast with a discourse on the city. The *stato* is about what happens outside the walls of the city, that is, outside the vivere civile.

18 Ibid., 171.

19 Pocock, *The Machiavellian Moment*, 53.

20 Brown, "De-masking Renaissance Republicanism," 183.

21 Quoted in Bullard, *Lorenzo il Magnifico*, 75. The Italian reads as

follows: "Che a questi tempi le cose sono giudicate piuttosto dagli effetti che dalle parole." My translation.

22 Ibid., 76.

23 Trexler, *Public Life in Renaissance Florence*, 339.

24 Ibid.

25 The *sacre rappresentazioni* (sing. *sacra rappresentazione*) (literally "sacred representations") were plays staged at festival time that enacted an event in the Bible. For a sustained theoretical treatment of the sacred and the festival, see Roger Caillois, *Man and the Sacred* and especially "The Sacred as Transgression: The Theory of the Festival," 97–127.

26 Richard Trexler, *Public Life in Renaissance Florence*, 340. The *"viva!"* is still shouted at Italian gatherings of all sorts (soccer matches and political rallies most notably), and its slogan is written in the shape of the double *V* (representing the two consonants in the word "viva"), found throughout Italian cities in the form of graffiti on billboards and public walls. Double *V* or "doppia vu" is the Italian pronunciation of the English letter *W*, but the symbol for the "viva" is inscribed as two *V*s crossing themselves in the middle. Also literally meaning "life," its negative or "down with" or "death with" equivalent is the upside down double *V*.

27 Ibid.

28 Conspirators, including members of the Pazzi family and Pope Sixtus IV, devised a plot to remove Lorenzo and his brother Giuliano from power in Florence. The Pazzi Conspiracy, if effective, would have placed the pope's nephew Girolamo Riario in power, adding the Florentine state to papal territorial holdings. On April 26, Giuliano de' Medici was assassinated during mass at the cathedral, while Lorenzo escaped. Although the Medici successfully quelled the conspiracy, revolts against their rule continued until the 1490s, when they were expelled from Florence (1494).

29 *Magnificenza alla corte dei Medici*.

30 Bullard, *Lorenzo il Magnifico*, 11. On the role of the circulation of coins as a technique of image making, see Kevin Sharpe's essay "An Image Dotting Rabble."

31 Orvieto, "Carnevale e Feste Fiorentine del tempo di Lorenzo de' Medici," 118.

32 Ventrone, "Lorenzo's *Politica Festiva*," 107. Also see Ventrone, "Feste e spettacoli nella Firenze di Lorenzo il Magnifico."

33 Carew-Reid, *Les fêtes florentines au temps de Lorenzo il Magnifico*, 6.

The original French reads: "Les festivités de la Florence du XVème siècle peuvent être interprétées comme une affirmation sociale doublée de la célébration du pouvoir en place. Elles furent de plus en plus tributaires de la personalité de ses dirigeants qui manipulèrent leurs éléments pour y gagner en prestige personnel." My translation.

34 See the Lorenzo de' Medici entries of the *Trionfi e canti carnascialeschi toscani del Rinascimento*.

35 Paola Ventrone, "Lorenzo's *Politica Festiva*," 107.

36 Konrad Eisenbichler, in an unpublished paper entitled "Sacred Plays and the Spectacle of Power in Florentine Confraternities," insists that to best understand Lorenzo's sacre rappresentazioni and how they were performed by the confraternities in the period, one cannot rely on the linguistic and textual aspect of the plays. Rather, one must pay attention to their status as part of feste, and thus must pay attention to the relationship between spectacle and power therein. Specifically, Eisenbichler (citing the accounts of Bartolomeo Masi) notes that one must "question the impact of the verbal text on an early-modern audience of adults because even those contemporary descriptions of theatrical performances that were jotted down by intelligent, learned adults, fail to note the content of the plays they mention, let alone indicate the play's 'message'."

37 The etymological origin of carnival from "*carnevale*" is a contraction of "*carne levale*," or without meat, referring to the period prior to Lent when one is permitted indulgences like excessive eating (hence our contemporary mardi gras or "Fat Tuesday"—the day before Ash Wednesday). The Lent period is a period of mourning and abstention intended to recall the forty days and forty nights Jesus passed in the desert prior to his triumphal entry into Jerusalem on Palm Sunday, culminating in the rituals of the Holy Week that include Good Friday and end with Easter Sunday. Carnival permits carnal indulgence all the while recalling the necessity of abstention (and the paschal sacrifice) to redeem one's concupiscence. After all, the point of the paschal sacrifice—Christ's crucifixion—is to redeem the sins of *carne* (the flesh). In carnival, the liminal scene of life and death is played out as a confrontation between the body and the soul through injunctions on the stomach. This, of course, is related to an entire tradition of alimentary and corporal metaphorics of what Ernst Robert Curtis calls "the palate of the mind." *European Literature and the Latin Middle Ages*, 136.

38 Camille, *Image on the Edge*, 70.

39 Bruscagli, *Trionfi e canti carnascialeschi toscani del Rinascimento*, xi. The original Italian reads: "Il 'tiranno' del Savonarola, suggestivamente distinto anche dalla richezza del suo guardaroba, non è qui soltanto l'*auctor* che segue con paterna affezione l'*iter* delle sue creature: è il signore che controlla lo svolgimento di una festa preordinata, che regola dall'interno, e in prima persona, l'uso di categorie 'popolari', in senso linguistico e sociologico, di cui egli è il primo e paradossale produttore." My translation.

40 Among the many important studies on the history of marginalia and the materiality of print culture, Michael Camille's *Image on the Edge* argues that a substantive shift occurred in the medieval understanding of textuality: "Once the manuscript page becomes a matrix of visual signs and is no longer one of flowing linear speech," he states, "the stage is set not only for supplementation and annotation but also for disagreement and juxtaposition—what the scholastics called *disputatio*." *Image on the Edge*, 21. See also H. J. Jackson, *Marginalia*.

41 Massumi, "Chaos in the 'Total Field' of Vision" in *Parables for the Virtual*, 145.

42 Without going into too much detail, Brunelleschi's experiment involved him standing in front of the baptistery in Florence's Piazza Duomo, holding a mirror with a hole drilled in it. The result of this experiment, as described by Samuel Y. Edgerton in *The Renaissance Rediscovery of Linear Perspective*, is that it showed "a geometric construction which could give a sense of unity and consistency to any illusionary plane" (129). Unfortunately, Brunelleschi's picture panels that resulted from these optical experiments have been lost.

43 Ibid., 10.

44 Ibid., 137.

45 In his introduction to *The Prince*, David Wootton helpfully points out that Brunelleschi is the only artist that Machiavelli cites in his works.

46 For a detailed account of Augustine and extromissive vision, see Eugene Vance's essay, "Seeing God: Augustine, Sensation, and the Mind's Eye."

47 Camille, "Before the Gaze," 207.

48 Ibid., 209.

49 Ibid., 200.

50 Vatter, *Between Form and Event*, 137–93.

51 Ibid., 182.

52 In *Machiavelli*, 927–31.

53 Larosa, "Autobiografia e tradizione letteraria nella 'Giornata' di Niccolò Machiavelli."

54 Ibid., 255. The original Italian reads: "in questa prospettiva i due tipi di lettura compiuti da Machiavelli, quello diurno e quello notturno, devono essere analizzati parallelamente, pur nella diversità degli intenti che li contradistinguono." My translation.

55 Machiavelli to Vettori, December 10, 1513, in *Machiavelli*, 929.

56 Peter Godman, *From Poliziano to Machiavelli: Florentine Humanism in the High Renaissance*, 257.

57 Machiavelli to Vettori, December 10, 1513, in *Machiavelli*, 929.

58 I would also note a further inversion to this basic dyad where illumination occurs at night and degradation during the day.

59 In his chapter on "Banquet Imagery" in *Rabelais and His World*, Bakhtin is explicit about this: "Eating and drinking are one of the most significant manifestations of the grotesque body. The distinctive character of this body is its open unfinished nature, its interaction with the world. These traits are most fully and concretely revealed in the act of eating; the body transgresses here its own limits: it swallows, devours, rends the world apart, is enriched and grows at the world's expense" (281).

60 Foucault, "Technologies of the Self" in *The Essential Foucault*, 145–69; see especially Foucault's treatment of Marcus Aurelius's letter to Fronto (AD 144–45) and its depiction of everyday life (gargling, eating, bathing) as part of the *souci de soi* (care of the self), 154.

61 For more on the role of ambivalence, renewal, and regeneration as sources of the early-modern cosmology of the vita festiva see Mikhail Bakhtin's discussion of ritual feast, the change of seasons, and the play of time in *Rabelais and His World*, 81–83.

62 Skinner, *Foundations of Modern Political Thought*, 128–29.

63 Machiavelli, *The Prince*, trans. Thompson, 45. The Italian is from *Il principe e altre opere politiche*, 67–69, and reads as follows: "Per tanto a uno principe è necessario sapere bene usare la bestia e lo uomo."

64 Machiavelli, *The Prince*, trans. Thompson, 46. The Italian reads: "essere gran simulatore e dissimulatore."

65 Ibid., 47. The Italian reads: "E li uomini in universali iudicano più alli occhi che alle mani; perché tocca a vedere a ognuno, a sentire a pochi." Not to be overlooked in this passage is the religious overtone referring us to the figure of the "doubting Thomas" (recounted in John 20:26–31) whose feast is celebrated on the second Sunday after Easter

and masterfully depicted in Caravaggio's *Doubting Thomas* (ca. 1602). I should add, as an aside which cannot be developed fully here, that in this and other paintings Caravaggio's "glance is a gesture of pointing" (Marin, *To Destroy Painting*, 164) that results in a kind of visual touching. What Caravaggio accomplished according to Marin's brilliant reading is quite simply the act of exposing mimesis as "an effect to be imprinted on the viewer's sensibility" (157) rather than mimesis understood as a representational structure of versimilitude. In this sense, intromission denies allegory its force by attributing the force of conviction to the gesture of impression.

66 For a more sustained engagement with Machiavelli's *ars rhetorica*, see Victoria Kahn, *Machiavellian Rhetoric*, especially part 1.

Chapter Four

Epigraph from Hume, *A Treatise of Human Nature*, book 1, part 4 ("Of Personal Identity"), section 6, paragraph 4.

1 *The Ring*, directed by Gore Verbinski; *The Ring Two*, directed by Hideo Nakata; *Ringu*, directed by Hideo Nakata.

2 Suzuki, *The Ring*, 146.

3 For a full explanation of the "irrational cut," see Deleuze, *Cinema 2*, 200–201; and Connolly, *Neuropolitics*, 135.

4 I should emphasize that this is the story as recounted in the novel. In the film, the rape and infection narrative is entirely omitted.

5 Suzuki, *The Ring*, 281.

6 Ibid., 177.

7 Marin, *To Destroy Painting*. See especially part 2, "Et in Arcana hoc."

8 Ibid., 105. Emphasis in original.

9 Marin, *To Destroy Painting*, 163.

10 I trust the reader to appreciate the extent to which my polemical assertions throughout this chapter stem from a profound indebtedness to those writers that traverse the boundaries of political theory and visual studies.

11 See Fried's discussion of the nonsubsumptive dialectic between the horizontal plane of representation (writing) and the vertical plane of representation (painting) in Thomas Eakins's *The Gross Clinic* in *Realism, Writing, Disfiguration*, especially 70–89.

12 In their own ways, I see all three of these thinkers sharing in a

critique of dialectical reason (and specifically, Hegel's view of history) as that mode of reasoning that insists on subsumption. Deleuze is most intensely committed to this critical project, to what he calls "the banality of the negative" (*Difference and Repetition*, 51—see also my *The Poetics of Political Thinking*, chapter 2), but so is Michael Fried's idea of a "non-subsumptive dialectic" and his discussion of the permanent revolution of self-criticism of modernist art (see *Realism, Writing, Disfiguration*; and "Three American Painters"). Not to be overlooked in this respect are Michel Foucault's lectures on Manet that emphasize Manet's discovery of the painting as object through the interplay of spectator, illumination, and the materiality of the canvas. See Foucault, *La peinture de Manet*.

13 Marin, *To Destroy Painting*, 108.

14 Fried, "Thoughts on Caravaggio."

15 Deleuze, *Francis Bacon*, 9.

16 Marin, *To Destroy Painting*, 106.

17 On the importance of "patina" to painting, see Brandi, *Teoria del restauro*, as well as Orlandi, "Il concetto di 'patina' nella *Teoria del restauro* di Cesare Brandi."

18 Marin, *To Destroy Painting*, 142.

19 Ibid., 143.

20 Ibid., 156.

21 Fried, "Thoughts on Caravaggio," 22.

22 The relationship between the paintbrush and the pen is explored once again and in a different context in Fried's *Realism, Writing, Disfiguration* as well as his *Courbet's Realism*.

23 This claim speaks to the strong Wittgensteinian strain in (especially) Fried's thought. See his discussion of conviction and convention in Wittgenstein's *Remarks on the Foundations of Mathematics* in "An Introduction to My Art Criticism," 31, but also his discussion of the art critic as a moral critic in part 1 of his "Three American Painters."

24 Marin, *To Destroy Painting*, 163.

25 Fried, *Absorption and Theatricality*. As of late, Fried has extended this analysis even further to include recent "documentary" photography (specifically the work of Jeff Wall), where he sees "a documentary look and an absorptive dramaturgy, [that coexist] with a foregrounding of the apparatus and a radical acknowledgment of the roles of both photographer and beholder." "Being There," 53–54. See also his most recent work in "Barthes's *Punctum*"; "Without a Trace"; and "Jeff Wall, Wittgenstein, and the Everyday."

26 Fried, "Thoughts on Caravaggio," 23. Emphasis in original.

27 Fried, *Absorption and Theatricality*, 118.

28 Ibid., 131. It is noteworthy that in a footnote Fried connects such phantasmagoric remarks to cinema (n. 78, p. 234) and especially to Stanley Cavell's work on cinema, *The World Viewed*.

29 And, as I argued in chapter 1, I also take this to be the point of Kant's antinormative stance vis-à-vis aesthetic judgment, exploited in his commitment to a disinterested interest in the appraisal of beauty.

30 Deleuze, *Francis Bacon*, 6. The elision of figuration is also crucial to Fried's readings of Jackson Pollock's *Out of the Web* (1949) and that work's success in at once restoring and "liberating the line from the task of figuration." Fried, "Three American Painters," 229. Given that Deleuze cites Fried's essay in the last pages of his book on Francis Bacon, one wonders about the extent to which Fried's account of Pollock influenced Deleuze's account of Bacon. Figure is capitalized here and throughout in order to remain consistent with Deleuze's use of this term and his distinction between "Figure" and "figuration" in chapter 1 of his *Francis Bacon*.

31 Deleuze, *Francis Bacon*, 48.

32 *Study after Velazquez's Portrait of Pope Innocent X* (1953) shows the image of a screaming Pope sitting on a chair. Due to the Bacon estate's restrictions on reproduction of images, I was not able to reproduce a version of that painting here. Readers interested in viewing this painting can go to the following web site: www.artquotes.net / masters / bacon / paint_study.htm (accessed July 12, 2008).

33 Deleuze, *Francis Bacon*, 36.

34 In this regard Deleuze asserts that "the body exerts itself in a very precise manner, or waits to escape from itself in a very precise manner. It is not I who attempts to escape from my body, it is the body that attempts to escape from itself by means of . . . in short, a spasm: the body as plexus, and its effort or waiting for a spasm." *Francis Bacon*, 15. Ellipsis in original.

35 Ibid., 40.

36 Deleuze also describes this phenomenon as the "Body-without-Organs." See my discussion of this in chapter 5.

37 Ibid., 34.

38 Deleuze, "Bartleby; or, The Formula." I take the force of Deleuze's reading of Bartleby to be the idea of a formula that undoes formalism. But this insight, I think, is also available in the approach to painting by both Fried and Marin, who are intensely interested in

artworks that, through formal techniques relevant to the enterprise of painting, at once undo themselves and the formal parameters of the painting itself. This is the moment of self-referentiality of these paintings and that makes, on Fried's account (especially), modernist paintings a "genre." What is relevant to them, in other words, is what he calls their moment of a "perpetual revolution—perpetual because bent on an unceasing radical self-criticism of themselves." "Three American Painters," 218.

39 The most extensive treatment of this is in chapter 14 of *Francis Bacon*, "Painters Recapitulate the History of Painting in Their Own Way." Here, Deleuze explains the origin of the concept in his readings of Aloïs Riegl's nineteenth-century writings on monuments in Riegl, "The Modern Cult of Monuments."

40 Marks, *The Skin of the Film*, 163.

41 Ibid.

42 Massumi, *Parables for the Virtual*, 170.

43 Suzuki, *The Ring*, 146.

44 For the purposes of this chapter, I will focus on the American version of the movie directed by Gore Verbinski, 2002.

45 Rancière, *La fable cinématographique*, 19. "Ses procédures d'art," Rancière states, "doivent construire des dramaturgies qui contrarient ses pouvoirs naturels. De sa nature technique à sa vocation artistique, la ligne n'est past droite. La fable cinématographique est une fable contrariée." (Cinema's artistic procedures construct dramas that thwart (or interrupt) its natural powers. The line from its technical nature to its artistic vocation is not a straight one. The cinematic fable is a contrarian one.) My translation.

46 Marin, *To Destroy Painting*, 105.

47 Stanley Cavell's early work on the ontology of film and the dynamics of audience and screen is relevant here. See especially the chapter "Photograph and Screen," in *The World Viewed* and his discussion of the difference between the screen and the frame (24).

48 The dynamics of immersion and viewing are introduced in the film through the simultaneity of the visual, tactile, and aural dimensions of the ring.

49 "Samara" is the American counterpart to the Japanese Sadako.

50 Suzuki, *The Ring*, 146.

51 Deleuze, *Francis Bacon*, 74.

52 Fried, *Courbet's Realism*, 269. See also Fried's discussion of near-

ness in the painting *An After Dinner at Ornans* (p. 87) and, most notably, his brief but illuminating analysis of the leg of the chair in that painting.

53 Suzuki, *The Ring*, 146. See also the discussion in chapter 1 of Kantian immediacy.

54 Cavell, *The World Viewed*, 105.

55 Mast, *Film / Cinema / Movie*, 56.

56 Ibid., 113. My emphasis.

57 As Lev Manovich shows in *The Language of New Media*, the printed word is only one out of three (or more) possible practices of cultural interface that modern viewing subjects must at once endure and negotiate.

58 On an earlier and not unrelated formulation of the viewing subject, see Vivian Sobchak's *The Address of the Eye*.

59 Rancière, Thesis 8 in "Ten Theses on Politics."

60 Connolly, "The Evangelical-Capitalist Resonance Machine," 871.

Chapter Five

Epigraph taken from *The Gay Science*, Book I, Section 7, p. 81.

1 Because I have chosen to focus on the place of flavor in political reflection, I will leave aside a third partition: the mouth as sexual organ—both expressive and consumptive in its orientation.

2 Some of these issues were first explored by the anthropologist Sidney Mintz who, in such works as *Sweetness and Power* and *Tasting Food, Tasting Freedom*, argues for the political relevance of food as a communicative practice. Furthermore, Jürgen Habermas inadvertently emphasizes the gustatory dimensions of the mouth when discussing the ale and coffee houses in the rise of the bourgeois public sphere. He does not, however, expand on the relevance of flavor and the palate of the mind in *The Structural Transformation of the Bourgeois Public Sphere*. I would like to thank a blind reviewer of Duke University Press for reminding me of this point.

3 Louis Marin, *Food for Thought*, 36.

4 For a compelling historical account of the theological implications of this distinction, see Camporesi's "The Stupendous Excess" and "In the Pit of the Stomach" in *The Fear of Hell*. The original Italian title is *La casa dell'eternità*.

5 Camporesi, "Introduzione," xxii.

6 Plato, *Republic*, 218.

7 Ibid., 217.

8 Ibid., 218–19.

9 Ibid., 222.

10 Sissa, *Il piacere e il male*, 42. The Italian reads as follows: "Per Platone, l'origine del disordine e della proliferazione delle passioni è quindi alimentare. È attraverso la bocca che gli uomini si lasciano attirare nella storia. È l'appetito che non soltanto determina l'avvento della mutazione, il cambiamento della città perfetta immaginaria, ma provoca anche le trasformazioni di un tipo di regime in un altro." My translation.

11 On Kant, freedom, and the experiential life see Guyer, *Kant and the Experience of Freedom*.

12 Kant, *Critique of Judgment*, 54 (div. 1, sec. 5). As mentioned earlier in this book, this and subsequent citations are taken from the Oxford translation.

13 Ibid.

14 Ibid.

15 As an aside, Kant's example corresponds to the modern dictum to not go grocery shopping when hungry.

16 Rousseau, "Discourse on the Origin of Inequality," 27.

17 See my treatment of Hobbes's *nosce teipsum* and its relation to his science of politics in *The Poetics of Political Thinking*, 19–25.

18 Rousseau, "Discourse on the Origin of Inequality," 33–34.

19 This, in fact, takes place through the performative utterance "this is mine," the transubstantiating incantation that marks the beginning of the second part of Rousseau's treatise. The "this is mine" is not simply the institution of property, it is an act of framing, the discovery that there is a "mine" that is at once one's property and one's propriety, it is testament to the imagination's capacity to invent possible worlds, and, ultimately, it marks the institution of authority, of a self who can speak as if there were a "this" to possess.

20 Ibid., 35.

21 Wingrove, *Rousseau's Republican Romance*, 59.

22 Rousseau, *Emile: Or, On Education*, book 1, n. 1.

23 Rousseau, *The Government of Poland*, 19.

24 Spang, *The Invention of the Restaurant*, 35.

25 Ibid., 36.

26 Ibid., 39.

27 Ibid., 63. Spang describes how "a restaurant meal also allowed others to be like Rousseau. With its private rooms, intimate tables, and particularized service, the restaurant made isolation available to

everybody. . . . The restaurant introduced Rousseau's desire into the marketplace."

28 Rousseau, "Discourse on the Origin of Inequality," 81.

29 Schlosser, *Fast Food Nation*, 123. To this end, one could make the claim that the first recorded act of moral transgression is a culinary one—the eating of the fruit from the tree of knowledge—which is subsequently reprised and restored at the last supper: the tear that Adam and Eve ensured by eating the apple that, according to Augustine, is the source of original sin and ultimately of humanity's discordant distanciation from the divine (see *Confessions*, book 8), is sutured by the paschal sacrifice, as recounted in the New Testament Gospels (see especially Matthew 26:26–29). In the case of Genesis (3:1–24), eating provokes both a literal and a figurative indigestion, a dissensual experience so powerful that a reconfiguration of Adam's and Eve's regime of perception occurs, forcing them to acknowledge each other's nakedness, and through that acknowledgment, experience shame. Like the ideal of the restaurant, the last supper narrative insists on the restorative aspect of eating; the sharing of the meal not only restores humanity to God's favor but it also encourages proper circulation; it is, in short, restorative of one's delicate (in this case, spiritual) constitution.

30 I attended the symposium which was held on March 15, 2004.

31 This debate is a version of the authenticity debates occurring in international courts and at G8 summits regarding the branding and production of indigenous food products.

32 "Al dente" refers to the texture of the pasta when it is cooked to the liminal point of being at once done and somewhat raw. Literally meaning "to the tooth," pasta cooked "al dente" means that it is still slightly crunchy when bitten into, leaving that recognizable slit of whiteness in the middle.

33 My point is that Barthes's connotative and denotative linguistic description of "Italianicity" in "The Rhetoric of the Image" cannot account for flavor as part of the visual experience. Thus, the moment that "al dente" enters into considerations of the condition of phenomenal perception, Barthes's semiotic account is disrupted. To use his own terms developed later in his career, the "al dente" flavor and texture here counts as the *punctum* of the experience of pasta. For his discussion of photography's punctum, see Barthes, *Camera Lucida*.

34 It goes without saying that this is, indeed, a bittersweet alliance given that Barilla's principal preoccupation was with access to North American market shares dominated by Catelli and other non-Italian

companies (and, it should be noted, I do not believe that Barilla was motivated by altruism in its efforts to educate taste). This is an especially relevant point to make given the political unrest during the ALMA conference, occurring, as it did, at the height of the Parmalat embezzlement scandal (Barilla and Parmalat are among the largest food manufacturers in Italy and both are indigenous to Parma, which is twenty kilometers from Colorno). See Povoledo, "Food School Opening Distracts from Parma Scandal."

35 The Italian history of appetite has been explored in recent studies written by a group of scholars primarily associated with the Università di Bologna including Paolo Sorcinelli in *Gli Italiani e il cibo*, as well as Alberto Capatti and Massimo Montanari in *Italian Cuisine*.

36 Carol Helstosky, *Garlic and Oil*, 14.

37 Ibid., 28.

38 Artusi, *Science in the Kitchen and the Art of Eating Well*, 115.

39 Ibid., 326.

40 Camporesi, "Introduzione," lix. See also Camporesi's "Bourgeois Cooking in the Nineteenth Century: Between Tradition and Renewal." The original Italian reads as follows: "la cucina dei 'signori' divulgata e democratizzata." My translation.

41 Importantly, as Capatti and Montanari point out in *Italian Cuisine*, "the adjective *raffinato* (refined) is often used, along with *delicato* (delicate) and *signorile* (elegant), to designate the style of the dishes, the choice of seasonings, and the distinctiveness of the flavors" (28).

42 Honig, *Democracy and the Foreigner*, 29.

43 The connection to Kant is mine, though the exposition of the triad is Camporesi's in his "Introduzione," xxxi.

44 Helstosky, *Garlic and Oil*, 132.

45 Schlosser, *Fast Food Nation*, 139.

46 Stille, "Slow Food."

47 Perillo, "Slowfood."

48 Petrini, *Slow Food*, xxiii.

49 Connolly, "Democracy and Time."

50 Slow Food's symbol is the snail, which is also the name of its newsletter. For more information see: www.slowfood.com.

51 Coles, "Moving Democracies."

52 Ibid., 695.

53 Petrini, *Slow Food*, 12.

54 Ibid., 13.

55 Ibid.

56 Ibid., 15.

57 Ibid., 17–18.

58 For a similar interpretation of the durational dimension of "slow food," see Berlant, "Slow Death (Sovereignty, Obesity, Lateral Agency)." For a more critical perspective on the Slow Food movement, see Meneley, "Extra-Virgin Olive Oil and Slow Food."

59 This particularist ethos is cognate with a political theorizing that, Linda Zerilli explains, "would turn on the ability to form critical judgments from within the ordinary, that is, on the reflective ability to relate particulars to each other in unexpected (not necessary or logical) ways by creating new forms of organizing our experience." Zerilli, *Feminism and the Abyss of Freedom*, 63.

60 Pollan, "Cruising on the Ark of Taste."

61 Ibid.

62 Petrini, *Slow Food*, 40.

63 Deleuze and Guattari, *A Thousand Plateaus*, 158. Deleuze reaffirms this point in his *Francis Bacon*, "In fact, the body without organs does not lack organs, it simply lacks the organism, that is, this particular organization of organs. The body without organs is thus defined by an indeterminate organ, whereas the organism is determined by determinate organs"(41).

64 Deleuze and Guattari, *A Thousand Plateaus*, 159.

65 For a compelling consideration of the writings of Gilles Deleuze and the culinary arts, see Rick Dolphijn's essay, "An Aesthetics of the Mouth."

66 This is an extension of my argument regarding Deleuze's debt to Kant in chapter 1.

67 Marin, *Food for Thought*, 36.

68 Foucault, *Dits et Ecrits, 1954–1988*. See especially vol. 4, 353–65 (the 1982 lectures at the Collège de France).

Epilogue

Epigraph from de Certeau, "The Madness of Vision," 25.

1 Hersh, "Torture at Abu Ghraib."

2 The Taguba Report is a report on the institutional failures of the Army prison system presented by Major General Antonio M. Taguba that was originally not intended for public release.

3 Hersh, "Torture at Abu Ghraib." Most recently, in the March 24, 2008 issue of *The New Yorker*, Philip Gourevitch and Errol Morris discuss how the person responsible for the photos taken at Abu Ghraib, Sabrina Harman, always wanted to become a forensic photographer and that by taking those candid photographs she imagined herself producing an exposé of what she felt was reprehensible conduct. See Gourevitch and Morris, "Annals of War."

4 Hersh, "Torture at Abu Ghraib."

5 This, ultimately, is the potential failure that resides in any gesture, claim, or image: the risk, that is, that it might not register attention.

6 Barthes, *Camera Lucida*, 27.

7 Ibid., 19.

8 My thinking on an ethics of appearance is indebted to Michael Fried's work on modern practices of beholding (with regards to Roland Barthes's work on photography, see especially Fried, "Barthes's *Punctum*"). Peter Nyers's discussion of "visualizing refugeeness" in *Rethinking Refugees,* 13–18 is also helpful. Here Nyers is concerned with the content (or, more precisely, a lack thereof) of humanitarian practices of representing refugeeness (like those found on the United Nations High Commissioner for Refugees Web site). My concern is less with the idea of content than with the fact that the images and photographs Nyers discusses mark an appearance of the refugee as a subjectivity that compels perceptual attention. The question from my perspective is not the nature and practice of representation per se but the partitions of perception that make the perceptibility of the refugee possible.

9 The word "monstrance" comes from Nancy, *The Ground of the Image*, 20–26, who, in turn, borrows it from Kacem, *Esthétique du chaos*.

10 For a cognate treatment of the Abu Ghraib photographs, also see Hariman and Lucaites, *No Caption Needed*, 291–301.

11 In *Administration of Torture*, Singh and Jaffer use ACLU and governmental documents to show that the abuse of prisoners is a matter of policy in U.S. detention facilities in Iraq, Afghanistan, and at Guantánamo Bay.

12 As Morton Schoolman shows in his work on the motility of aesthetic objects, appearances have a palpability about them that is available regardless of a structure of belief that might either justify them or give them a meaning. See especially Schoolman, "The Next Enlightenment."

13 Manovich, *The Language of New Media*, 117.

BIBLIOGRAPHY

Arendt, Hannah. *The Human Condition*. Chicago, Ill.: University of Chicago Press, 1958.

——. *Hannah Arendt: The Recovery of the Public World*. Ed. Melvyn A. Hill. New York: St. Martin's Press, 1979.

——. *Eichmann in Jerusalem: A Report on the Banality of Evil*. New York: Penguin Classics, 1994.

——. *Responsibility and Judgment*. New York: Schocken Books, 2005.

Artusi, Pellegrino. *La scienza in cucina e l'arte di mangiar bene*. Torino: Einaudi, 1970.

——. *Science in the Kitchen and the Art of Eating Well*. Trans. Murtha Baca. Toronto: University of Toronto Press, 2003.

Augustine. *Confessions*. Trans. Henry Chadwick. London: Oxford University Press, 1998.

Bakhtin, Mikhail. *Rabelais and His World*. Trans. Hélène Iswolsky. Bloomington: Indiana University Press, 1984.

——. *Speech Genres and Other Late Essays*. Trans. Vern W. McGee. Austin: University of Texas Press, 1989.

——. "The Problem of Speech Genres." In Bakhtin, *Speech Genres and Other Late Essays*, 60–102.

Barthes, Roland. *Camera Lucida: Reflections on Photography*. Trans. Richard Howard. New York: Hill and Wang, 1982.

——. *Image, Music, Text*. Trans. Stephen Heath. New York: Hill and Wang, 1988.

——. "The Grain of the Voice." In Barthes, *Image, Music, Text*, 179–89.

——. "The Rhetoric of the Image." In Barthes, *Image, Music, Text*, 32–51.

Bassi, Rafaella. "Chioschi: Appunti di storia e di quotidianità." *Arredo & Città* 2 (September 1988): 28–31.

Bataille, Georges. *The Accursed Share: An Essay on General Economy*. Vol. 1. Trans. Robert Hurley. New York: Zone, 1988.

——. *The Bataille Reader.* Fred Botting and Scott Wilson, eds. Oxford: Blackwell, 1997.

——. "The Notion of Expenditure." In Bataille, *The Bataille Reader*, 167–81.

Bazzani, Marco. "Un mini-museo d'arte." *La Cronaca di Cremona*, February, 2004.

Bentham, Jeremy. *Bentham's Theory of Fictions*. Ed. C. K. Ogden. London, UK: Kegan Paul, Trench, Trübner, 1932.

Berlant, Lauren. "Slow Death (Sovereignty, Obesity, Lateral Agency)." *Critical Inquiry* 33:4 (summer 2007): 754–80.

Bible, The: Authorized King James Version with Apocrypha. Oxford: Oxford University Press, 1997.

Bolsi, Franco Giuseppe. "Acanto." In *Il grande fiume* (Casalmaggiore, Italy), summer, 2003, 18.

Brandi, Cesare. *Teoria del restauro.* Milano: Einaudi, 1977.

Brown, Alison. "De-masking Renaissance Republicanism." In *Renaissance Humanism: Reappraisals and Reflections*, 129–99. Ed. James Hankins. Cambridge: Cambridge University Press, 2000.

Bruscagli, Riccardo. *Trionfi e canti carnascialeschi toscani del Rinascimento.* Roma: Salerno, 1986.

Bullard, Melissa. *Lorenzo il Magnifico: Image and Anxiety, Politics and Finance.* Firenze: Leo S. Olschki Editore, 1994.

Burckhardt, Jacob. *The Civilization of the Renaissance in Italy*. Trans. S. G. C. Middlemore. N.Y: Penguin Classics, 1990.

Butler, Judith. "Endangered / Endangering: Schematic Racism and White Paranoia." In *The Butler Reader*, 204–11. Ed. Sara Salih. Malden, Mass.: Blackwell Publishing, 2004.

——. *Giving an Account of Oneself.* New York: Fordham University Press, 2005.

Caillois, Roger. *Man and the Sacred.* Urbana: University of Illinois Press, 2001.

Camille, Michael. *Image on the Edge: The Margins of Medieval Art.* London: Reaktion Books, 1992.

——. "Before the Gaze: The Internal Senses and Late Medieval Practices of Seeing." In *Visuality before the Renaissance*, 197–223. Ed. Robert S. Nelson. Cambridge: Cambridge University Press, 2000.

Camporesi, Piero. "Introduzione." In Pellegrino Artusi, *La scienza in cucina e l'arte di mangiar bene*, xv–lxxviii. Torino: Einaudi, 1970.

——. *La casa dell'eternità*. Milano: Garzanti Editore, 1987.
——. *Fear of Hell: Images of Damnation and Salvation in Early-Modern Europe*. University Park: Pennsylvania State University Press, 1991.
——. *The Magic Harvest*. Trans. J. K. H. Cambridge: Polity Press, 1998.
——. "Bourgeois Cooking in the Nineteenth Century: Between Tradition and Renewal." In Camporesi, *The Magic Harvest*, 113–52.
Capatti, Alberto, and Massimo Montanari. *Italian Cuisine: A Cultural History*. New York: Columbia University Press, 2003.
Carew-Reid, Nicole. *Les fêtes florentines au temps de Lorenzo il Magnifico*. Firenze: Leo S. Olschki Editore, 1995.
Cavell, Stanley. *The World Viewed*. Cambridge, Mass.: Harvard University Press, 1980.
Celes, Luciano. "Picture Battles in the Piazza: The Political Poster." In *The Art of Persuasion*, 124–79. Luciano Celes and Lucio Sponza, eds. New York: Manchester University Press, 2001.
Chartier, Roger. *The Order of Books*. Trans. Lydia G. Cochrane. Stanford, Calif.: Stanford University Press, 1994.
Coles, Romand. "Moving Democracies: Industrial Areas Foundation Social Movements and the Political Arts of Listening, Traveling, and Tabling." *Political Theory* 32 (October 2004): 678–705.
Connolly, William E. *Neuropolitics: Thinking, Culture, Speed*. Minneapolis: University of Minnesota Press, 2002.
——. "Democracy and Time." In Connolly, *Neuropolitics*, 140–75.
——. "The Evangelical-Capitalist Resonance Machine." *Political Theory* 33:6 (December 2005): 869–86.
Coole, Diana. *Merleau-Ponty and Modern Politics after Anti-Humanism*. New York: Rowman and Littlefield Publishers, 2007.
Cornell, Drucilla. *Defending Ideals*. New York: Routledge, 2004.
Crary, Jonathan. *Techniques of the Observer*. Cambridge, Mass.: MIT Press, 1992.
Curtis, Ernst Robert. *European Literature and the Latin Middle Ages*. Princeton, N.J.: Princeton University Press, 1973.
Danto, Arthur. *The Transfiguration of the Commonplace*. Cambridge, Mass.: Harvard University Press, 1981.
de Certeau, Michel. "The Madness of Vision." *Enclitic*7:1 (1983): 24–31.
——. *The Writing of History*. Trans. Tom Conley. New York: Columbia University Press, 1992.
——. "Vocal Utopias: Glossolalias." *Representations* 56 (autumn 1996): 29–57.
——. *The Practice of Everyday Life*. Trans. Timothy J. Tomasik. Minneapolis: University of Minnesota Press, 1998.

Dean, Jodi, ed. *Cultural Studies and Political Theory*. Ithaca, N.Y.: Cornell University Press, 2000.

Deleuze, Gilles. *Empiricism and Subjectivity: An Essay on Hume's Theory of Human Nature*. Trans. Constantin V. Boundas. New York: Columbia University Press, 1991.

——. *Kant's Critical Philosophy*. Trans. Hugh Tomlinson and Barbara Habberjam. Minneapolis: University of Minnesota Press, 1993.

——. *Difference and Repetition*. Trans. Paul Patton. New York: Columbia University Press, 1994.

——. *Cinema 2: The Time-Image*. Trans. Hugh Tomlinson. Minneapolis: University of Minnesota Press, 1997.

——. *Essays: Critical and Clinical*. Trans. Daniel W. Smith and Michael A. Greco. Minneapolis: University of Minnesota Press, 1997.

——. "Bartleby; or, The Formula." In Deleuze, *Essays: Critical and Clinical*, 68–90.

——. "To Have Done with Judgment." In Deleuze, *Essays: Critical and Clinical*, 126–35.

——. *Francis Bacon: The Logic of Sensation*. Trans. Daniel W. Smith. Minneapolis: University of Minnesota Press, 2004.

Deleuze, Gilles, and Félix Guattari. *A Thousand Plateaus: Capitalism and Schizophrenia*. Trans. Brian Massumi. Minneapolis: University of Minnesota Press, 1987.

Dolphijn, Rick. "An Aesthetics of the Mouth: Creativity Between the Culinary and the Arts." *Angelaki* 11:1 (April 2006): 179–88.

Don Camillo. Dir. Julien Duvivier. Francinex, 1951.

Dondi, Marco. "Piazzale Loreto." In *I luoghi della memoria: Simboli e miti dell'Italia Unita*, 487–99. Ed. Mario Isnenghi. Roma: Laterza, 1997.

Edgerton, Samuel Y. *The Renaissance Rediscovery of Linear Perspective*. New York: Harper and Row Publishers, 1976.

Edwards, Brent Hayes. "Louis Armstrong and the Syntax of Scat." *Critical Inquiry* 28:3 (spring 2002): 618–49.

Eisenbichler, Konrad. *Carnival and the Carnivalesque*. Konrad Eisenbichler and Wim Hüsken, eds. Atlanta, Ga.: Rodopi Press, 1999.

——. "Sacred Plays and the Spectacle of Power in Florentine Confraternities." Paper presented at the annual meeting of the Renaissance Society of America, Cambridge, UK, April 7–9, 2005.

Erasmus, Desiderius. *Praise of Folly*. Ware: Wordsworth Editions Limited, 1998.

Ferguson, Frances. *Pornography, the Theory*. Chicago, Ill.: University of Chicago Press, 2004.

Ferguson, Kennan. *The Politics of Judgment: Aesthetics, Identity, and Political Theory*. New York, N.Y.: Lexington Books, 2007.

Flaxman, Gregory, ed. *The Brain is the Screen: Deleuze and the Philosophy of Cinema*. Minneapolis: University of Minnesota Press, 2000.

Foucault, Michel. *Dits et Ecrits, 1954–1988*. Paris: Gallimard, 1994.

——. "Technologies of the Self." In *The Essential Foucault*, 145–69. Paul Rabinow and Nikolas Rose, eds. New York: New Press, 2003.

——. *La peinture de Manet*. Paris: Editions du Seuil, 2004.

——. *The Hermeneutics of the Subject: Lectures at the Collège de France, 1981–1982*. Ed. Frédéric Gros. New York: Picador, 2005.

Fried, Michael. *Absorption and Theatricality: Painting and Beholder in the Age of Diderot*. Los Angeles: University of California Press, 1980.

——. *Realism, Writing, Disfiguration*. Chicago, Ill.: University of Chicago Press, 1987.

——. *Courbet's Realism*. Chicago, Ill.: University of Chicago Press, 1990.

——. "Thoughts on Caravaggio." *Critical Inquiry* 24 (autumn 1997): 13–56.

——. *Art and Objecthood*. Chicago, Ill.: University of Chicago Press, 1998.

——. "Three American Painters: Noland, Olitski, Stella." In Fried, *Art and Objecthood*, 213–65.

——. "An Introduction to My Art Criticism." In Fried, *Art and Objecthood*, 1–74.

——. "Being There: Michael Fried on Two Pictures by Jeff Wall." *Artforum* 43 (September 2004): 53–54.

——. "Barthes's *Punctum*." *Critical Inquiry* 31 (spring 2005): 539–74.

——. "Without a Trace." *Artforum* 43 (March 2005): 198–203.

——. "Jeff Wall, Wittgenstein, and the Everyday." *Critical Inquiry* 33 (spring 2007): 495–526.

Garroni, Giovanni. *Elogio dell'imprecisione: Percezione e rappresentazione*. Torino: Bollati Boringhieri editore, s.r.1., 2005.

Ginzburg, Carlo. *The Cheese and the Worms*. Trans. John Tedeschi and Anne C. Tedeschi. Baltimore, Md.: Johns Hopkins University Press, 1992.

Godman, Peter. *From Poliziano to Machiavelli: Florentine Humanism in the High Renaissance*. Princeton, N.J.: Princeton University Press, 1998.

Gourevitch, Philip, and Errol Morris. "Annals of War: Exposure; The Woman behind the Camera at Abu Ghraib." *The New Yorker*, March 24, 2008.

Guillory, John. "The Memo and Modernity." *Critical Inquiry* 31 (fall 2004): 108–32.

Guyer, Paul. *Kant and the Experience of Freedom*. Cambridge: Cambridge University Press, 1996.

——. *Values of Beauty: Historical Essays in Aesthetics.* Cambridge: Cambridge University Press, 2005.

Habermas, Jürgen. *The Structural Transformation of the Public Sphere*. Trans. Thomas Burger and Frederick Lawrence. Cambridge, Mass.: MIT Press, 1991.

Hariman, Robert, and John Louis Lucaites. *No Caption Needed: Iconic Photographs, Popular Culture, and Liberal Democracy*. Chicago, Ill.: University of Chicago Press, 2007.

Helstosky, Carol. *Garlic and Oil: Food and Politics in Italy*. New York: Berg, 2004.

Hersh, Seymour M. "Torture at Abu Ghraib." *The New Yorker*, May 10, 2004.

Honig, Bonnie. *Democracy and the Foreigner*. Princeton, N.J.: Princeton University Press, 2003.

Hume, David. *A Treatise of Human Nature*. Oxford: Oxford University Press, 2000.

Huntington, Samuel P., "The Clash of Civilizations?" *Foreign Affairs* 72:3 (summer 1993): 21–49.

Hutcheson, Francis. *An Inquiry into the Original of Our Ideas of Beauty and Virtue*. Indianapolis, Ind.: Liberty Fund Inc., 2004.

Isnenghi, Mario. *L'Italia in piazza*. Milano: Arnold Mondadori Editori, 1994.

Jackson, H. J. *Marginalia: Readers Writing in Books*. New York: Metropolitan Museum of Art, 2002.

Kacem, Mehdi Belhaj.*Esthétique du chaos*.Auch: Tristram Editeurs, 2000.

Kahn, Victoria. *Machiavellian Rhetoric: From the Counter-Reformation to Milton*. Princeton, N.J.: Princeton University Press, 1994.

Kandinsky, Wassily. *Concerning the Spiritual in Art*. Trans. M. T. H. Sadler. New York: Dover, 1977.

——. *Point and Line to Plane.* Trans. Howard Dearstyne and Hilla Rebay. New York: Dover, 1979.

Kant, Immanuel. *Critique of Judgment*. Trans. James Creed Meredith. London: Oxford University Press, 2007.

——. *Critique of Judgment*. Trans. J. H. Bernard. New York: Prometheus Books, 2000.

Larosa, Stella. "Autobiografia e tradizione letteraria nella 'Giornata' di Niccolò Machiavelli." *Interpres* 22 (2003): 223–75.

Machiavelli, Niccolò. *Machiavelli: The Chief Works and Others*. Vol. 2. Trans. Allan Gilbert. Durham, N.C.: Duke University Press, 1989.

——. *The Prince*. Trans. N. H. Thompson. New York: Dover Publications, 1992.

——. *The Prince*. Trans. David Wootton. New York: Hackett Publishing Company, 1995.
——. *Il principe e altre opere politiche*. Milano: Garzanti, 2002.
Magnificenza alla corte dei Medici: Arte a Firenze alla fine del cinquecento. Catalogo della mostra, Firenze, Palazzo Pitti, Museo degli Argenti. Milano: Electa, 1997.
Manning, Erin. *Politics of Touch: Sense, Movement, Sovereignty*. Minneapolis: University of Minnesota Press, 2007.
Manovich, Lev. *The Language of New Media*. Cambridge, Mass.: MIT Press, 2001.
Marin, Louis. *Food for Thought*. Trans. Mette Hjort. Baltimore, Md.: Johns Hopkins University Press, 1989.
——. *To Destroy Painting*. Trans. Mette Hjort. Chicago, Ill.: University of Chicago Press, 1994.
Markell, Patchen. *Bound by Recognition*. Princeton, N.J.: Princeton University Press, 2003.
Marks, Laura. *The Skin of the Film*. Durham, N.C.: Duke University Press, 2000.
Massumi, Brian. *Parables for the Virtual: Movement, Affect, Sensation*. Durham, N.C.; Duke University Press, 2002.
——. "Chaos in the 'Total Field' of Vision." In Massumi, *Parables for the Virtual*, 144–61.
Mast, Gerald. *Film / Cinema / Movie: A Theory of Experience*. New York: Harper and Row Publishers, 1977.
Mauss, Marcel. *The Gift*. Trans. W. D. Halls. New York: Norton, 1990.
McCormick, John. "MACHIAVELLI AGAINST REPUBLICANISM: On the Cambridge School's 'Guicciardinian Moments'." *Political Theory* 31 (October 2003): 615–43.
McLuhan, Marshall. *Understanding Media: The Extensions of Man*. Toronto: Signet Books, 1966.
Meneley, Anne. "Extra-Virgin Olive Oil and Slow Food." *Anthropologica* 46 (2004): 165–76.
Merleau-Ponty, Maurice. *Sense & Non-Sense*. Evanston, Ill.: Northwestern University Press, 1964.
——. *Phenomenology of Perception*. New York, N.Y.: Routledge, 1996.
Michaels, Walter Benn. *The Shape of the Signifier.* Princeton, N.J.: Princeton University Press, 2004.
Mintz, Sydney. *Sweetness and Power: The Place of Sugar in Modern History*. New York: Penguin Books, 1986.

———. *Tasting Food, Tasting Freedom: Excursions into Eating, Power, and the Past.* Boston, Mass.: Beacon Press, 1996.

Morrone, M. Concetta, John Ross, and David Burr. "Saccadic eye movements cause compression of time as well as space." In *Nature Neuroscience* 8:7 (July 2005): 950–54.

Nancy, Jean-Luc. *Noli me tangere: Essai sur la levée du corps.* Paris: Bayard, 2003.

———. *The Ground of the Image.* Trans. Jeff Fort. New York: Fordham University Press, 2005.

Nietzsche, Friedrich. *The Gay Science.* Trans. Walter Kaufmann. New York: Vintage Books, 1974.

Nyers, Peter. *Rethinking Refugees: Beyond States of Emergency.* New York: Routledge, 2006.

Orlandi, Marco. "Il concetto di 'patina' nella *Teoria del restauro* di Cesare Brandi." PhD diss., Istituto per l'arte e il restauro, Palazzo Spinelli, Firenze, Italy, 1998.

———. *Edicola nel tempo.* Porretta Terme (Bologna): I quaderni del Battello Ebbro, 2001.

———. "L'arredo urbano: Il chiosco dei giornali di Piazza Garibaldi." In *L'Età progettuale—scienza, arte e industria a Casalmaggiore (1820–1911)*, 173–77. Ed. Valter Rosa. Casalmaggiore: Edizioni Biblioteca Civica A. E. Mortara.

Orvieto, Paolo. "Carnevale e Feste Fiorentine del tempo di Lorenzo de' Medici." In *Lorenzo il Magnifico e il suo tempo*, 161–88. Ed. Gian Carlo Garfagnini. Firenze: Leo S. Olschki Editore, 1992.

Oxford English Dictionary Online, The. 2nd ed. 1989. Oxford University Press.

Panagia, Davide, and Jacques Rancière. "Dissenting Words: A Conversation with Jacques Rancière." *Diacritics* 30 (summer 2000): 113–26.

———. "*The Shape of the Signifier* or, The Ontology of Argument." In *Theory and Event* 8:2 (2005): n.p.

———. *The Poetics of Political Thinking.* Durham, N.C.: Duke University Press, 2006.

Panofsky, Erwin. *Perspective as Symbolic Form.* Trans. Christopher Wood. Cambridge, Mass.: Zone Books, 1993.

Perillo, Davide. "Slowfood: Le buone idee sono bipartisan." *Corriere della Sera Magazine*, May 26, 2005.

Petrini, Carlo. *Slow Food: The Case for Taste.* Trans. William McCuaig. New York: Columbia University Press, 2004.

Plato. *Republic.* Trans. Benjamin Jowett. New York: Dover Publications, 2000.

Pocock, John G. A. *The Machiavellian Moment.* Princeton, N.J.: Princeton University Press, 2003.

Pollan, Michael. "Cruising on the Ark of Taste." *Motherjones.com* (May / June, 2003), http://www.motherjones.com/news/feature/2003/05/ma_372_01.html (accessed June 5, 2006).

Povoledo, Elisabetta. "Food School Opening Distracts from Parma Scandal." *International Herald Tribune*, March 16, 2004.

Pugliese, Olga Zorzi. "L'evoluzione della struttura dialogica nel *Libro del cortegiano*." In *Il sapere delle parole: Studi sul dialogo latino e italiano del Rinascimento*, 59–64. Walter Geerts, Annick Paternoster, and Franco Pignatti, eds. Roma: Bulzoni, 2001.

Radnóti, Sándor. *The Fake: Forgery and its Place in Art*. Trans. Ervin Dunai. New York: Rowman and Littlefield, 1999.

Rancière, Jacques. *The Names of History*. Trans. Hassan Melehy. Minneapolis: University of Minnesota Press, 1994.

——. *Dis-Agreement: Politics and Philosophy*. Trans. Julie Rose. Minneapolis: University of Minnesota Press, 1998.

——. *La fable cinématographique*. Paris: Editions du Seuil, 2001.

——. "Ten Theses on Politics." *Theory & Event* 5:3 (2001): n.p.

——. *The Flesh of Words*. Trans. Charlotte Mandell. Stanford, Calif.: Stanford University Press, 2004.

——. "Deleuze, Bartleby, and the Literary Formula." In Rancière, *The Flesh of Words*, 146–64.

——. *The Philosopher and His Poor*. Trans. Andrew Parker. Durham, N.C.: Duke University Press, 2004.

——. *The Politics of Aesthetics*. Trans. Gabriel Rockhill. New York: Continuum, 2004.

——. "Thinking between Disciplines: An Aesthetics of Knowledge." *Parrhesia* 1 (2006): 1–12.

Rawls, John. *Political Liberalism*. Cambridge, Mass.: Harvard University Press, 1993.

Ricoeur, Paul. *Time and Narrative*. Vol. 1. Trans. Kathleen McLaughlin and David Pellauer. Chicago, Ill.: University of Chicago Press, 1984.

Riegl, Aloïs. "The Modern Cult of Monuments: Its Character and Its Origin." *Oppositions* 25 (fall 1982): 21–51.

Ring, The. Dir. Gore Verbinski. Dreamworks, 2002.

Ring Two, The. Dir. Hideo Nakata. Dreamworks, 2005.

Ringu. Dir. Hideo Nakata. Kadokawa Shoten Publishing, 1998.

Rockhill, Gabriel. "The Silent Revolution." *SubStance* 33:1 (2004): 54–76.

Rodowick, David Norman. *Reading the Figural, or, Philosophy after the New Media*. Durham, N.C.: Duke University Press, 2001.

Romano, Marco. "Le piazze e i cittadini." *Corriere della Sera*, July 4, 2003.

Rousseau, Jean-Jacques. *The Government of Poland*. Trans. Willmoore Kendall. New York: Hackett, 1985.

——. *Basic Political Writings*. Trans. Donald A. Cress. New York: Hackett, 1987.

——. "Discourse on the Origin of Inequality." In Rousseau, *Basic Political Writings*, 25–110.

——. *Emile: Or, On Education*. Trans. Barbara Foxley. Project Gutenberg Online, Edition, http://www.gutenberg.org/dirs/etext04/emile10.txt (accessed June 6, 2008).

Saint-Exupéry, Antoine de. *Le Petit Prince*. New York: Harvest Books, 2000.

Sanga, Glauco. "Campane e campanili." In *I luoghi della memoria: Simboli e miti dell'Italia unita*, 29–45. Ed. Mario Isnenghi. Milano: Editori Laterza, 1996.

Sarno, Niccolo. "EU Chocolate Vote Threatens Cocoa Producers." *Third World Network*, http://www.twnside.org.sg/title/vote.htm (accessed June 5, 2008).

Saussure, Ferdinand de. *Course in General Linguistics*. Trans. Wade Baskin. New York: McGraw Hill, 1966.

Schlosser, Eric. *Fast Food Nation*. New York: Harper Perennial, 2005.

Schoolman, Morton, "The Next Enlightenment: Aesthetic Reason in Modern Art and Mass Culture." *Journal for Cultural Research* 9:1 (January 2005): 43–67.

Shapiro, Michael J. *Deforming American Political Thought: Ethnicity, Facticity, and Genre*. Lexington: University Press of Kentucky, 2006.

Sharpe, Kevin. "An Image Dotting Rabble: The Failure of Republican Culture in Seventeenth-Century England." In *Refiguring Revolutions*, 25–56. Kevin Sharpe and Steven N. Zwicker, eds. Los Angeles: University of California Press, 1998.

Shaviro, Steven.*The Cinematic Body*. Minneapolis: University of Minnesota Press, 1993.

——. "Beauty Lies in the Eye." In *A Shock to Thought: Expressions After Deleuze and Guattari*, 9–19.Ed. Brian Massumi. New York: Routledge University Press, 2002.

Silverman, Kaja. *The Threshold of the Visible World*. New York: Routledge, 1995

Singh, Amrit, and Jameel Jaffer. *Administration of Torture: A Documentary Record from Washington to Abu Ghraib and Beyond*. New York: Columbia University Press, 2007.

Sissa, Giulia. *Il piacere e il male: Sesso, droga, filosofia*. Milano: Feltrinelli, 1999.

Skinner, Quentin. "Meaning and Understanding in the History of Ideas." In Skinner, *Visions of Politics*. Vol. 1, *Regarding Method*. Originally published in *History and Theory* 8 (1969): 3–53.

———. *Foundations of Modern Political Thought*. Vol. 1, *The Renaissance*. Cambridge: Cambridge University Press, 1978.

———. *Visions of Politics*. Vol. 1, *Regarding Method*. Cambridge: Cambridge University Press, 2003.

———. "Interpretation and the Understanding of Speech Acts." In Skinner, *Visions of Politics*, 103–27.

Smith, Daniel W. "Deleuze's Theory of Sensation: Overcoming the Kantian Duality." In *Deleuze: A Critical Reader*, 29–56. Ed. Paul Patton. Oxford: Blackwell Publishers, 1996.

———. "Deleuze, Kant, and the Theory of Immanent Ideas." In *Deleuze and Philosophy*, 43–61. Ed. Constantine V. Boundas. Edinburgh: Edinburgh University Press, 2006. 43–61.

Sobchak, Vivian. *The Address of the Eye: A Phenomenology of Film Experience*. Princeton, N.J.: Princeton University Press, 1992.

———. *Carnal Thoughts: Embodiment and Moving Image Culture*. Los Angeles: University of California Press, 2004.

Sorcinelli, Paolo. *Gli Italiani e il cibo*. Bologna: CLUEB, 1992.

Spang, Rebecca. *The Invention of the Restaurant*. Cambridge, Mass.: Harvard University Press, 2001.

Stille, Alexander. "Slow Food." *The Nation*, August 9, 2001.

Strocchia, Sharon T. *Death and Ritual in Renaissance Florence*. Baltimore, Md.: Johns Hopkins University Press, 1992.

Struever, Nancy. *Theory as Practice*. Chicago, Ill.: University of Chicago Press, 1992.

Suzuki, Koji. *The Ring*. New York: Vertical Inc., 2004. Originally published in Japan as *Ringu*.

Tarnopolsky, Christina. "Platonic Reflections on the Aesthetic Dimensions of Deliberative Democracy." *Political Theory* 35 (2007): 288–312.

Taylor, Charles. "Interpretation and the Sciences of Man." In *Philosophy and the Human Sciences*, 15–57. New York: Cambridge University Press, 1985.

———. "The Politics of Recognition." In *Multiculturalism: Examining the Politics of Recognition*, 25–74. Ed. Amy Gutmann. Princeton, N.J.: Princeton University Press, 1994.

Trexler, Richard. *Public Life in Renaissance Florence*. Ithaca, N.Y.: Cornell University Press, 1991.

Vance, Eugene. "Seeing God: Augustine, Sensation, and the Mind's Eye." In

Rethinking the Medieval Senses, 1329. Stephen G. Nichols, Andreas Kablitz, and Alison Calhoun, eds. Baltimore, Md.: Johns Hopkins University Press, 2008. 13–29.

Vatter, Miguel. *Between Form and Event: Machiavelli's Theory of Political Freedom*. Boston, Mass.: Kluwer Academic Publishing, 2000.

Ventrone, Paola. "Feste e spettacoli nella Firenze di Lorenzo il Magnifico." In *Le tems revient, 'ltempo si rinuova*, 21–53. Firenze: Silvana Editoriale, 1992.

——. "Lorenzo's *Politica Festiva*." In *Lorenzo The Magnificent: Culture and Politics*, 105–16. Michael Mallet and Nicholas Mann, eds. London: The Warburg Institute, 1996.

Viroli, Maurizio. "Machiavelli and the Republican Idea of Politics." In *Machiavelli and Republicanism*, 143–72. Gisela Bock, Quentin Skinner, and Maurizio Viroli, eds. Cambridge: Cambridge University Press, 1990.

Warner, Michael. *Publics and Counterpublics*. New York: Zone Books, 2002.

White, Hayden. *Metahistory: The Historical Imagination in Nineteenth-Century Europe*. Baltimore, Md.: Johns Hopkins University Press, 1975.

Wingrove, Elizabeth. *Rousseau's Republican Romance*. Princeton, N.J.: Princeton University Press, 2000.

Wittgenstein, Ludwig. *Philosophical Investigations*. Trans. G. E. M. Anscombe. Oxford, UK: Basil Blackwell, 1976.

——. *Remarks on the Foundations of Mathematics*. Ed. Cora Diamond. Chicago, Ill.: University of Chicago Press, 1976.

Wolfe, Katharine. "From Aesthetics to Politics: Rancière, Kant and Deleuze." *Journal of Contemporary Aesthetics* 4 (2006): n.p.

Young, Iris Marion. *On Female Body Experience: "Throwing like a Girl" and Other Essays*. Oxford, UK: Oxford University Press, 2005.

Zerilli, Linda. *Feminism and the Abyss of Freedom*. Chicago, Ill.: University of Chicago Press, 2005.

Žižek, Slavoj. *The Sublime Object of Ideology*. New York: Verso, 1989.

——. *Looking Awry: An Introduction to Jacques Lacan through Popular Culture*. Cambridge, Mass.: MIT Press, 1992.

INDEX

DAVIDE PANAGIA is a political and cultural theorist who holds the Canada Research Chair in Cultural Studies. He is an associate professor in the Cultural Studies department at Trent University and the author of *The Poetics of Political Thinking*, also published by Duke University Press (2006).

Library of Congress Cataloging-in-Publication Data
Panagia, Davide, 1971–
The political life of sensation / Davide Panagia.
p. cm.
Includes bibliographical references and index.
ISBN 978-0-8223-4463-6 (cloth : alk. paper)
ISBN 978-0-8223-4479-7 (pbk. : alk. paper)
1. Senses and sensation—Political aspects.
2. Senses and sensation—Moral and ethical aspects.
3. Perception—Political aspects. 4. Perception—Moral and ethical aspects. I. Title.
BD214.P36 2009
121′.35—dc22 2008051836